THE CASANOVA SEXICON

OTHER BOOKS BY ERIC NICOL

Sense and Nonsense (Ryerson Press, 1947)

The Roving Eye (Ryerson Press, 1950)

Twice Over Lightly (Ryerson, Press, 1953)

Shall We Join the Ladies? (Ryerson Press, 1955)

Girdle Me A Globe (Ryerson Press, 1957)

An Uninhibited History of Canada [with Peter Whalley] (Musson, 1958)

In Darkest Domestica (Ryerson Press, 1959)

Say, Uncle (Ryerson Press, 1961)

A Herd of Yaks (Ryerson Press, 1962)

Russia, Anyone? [with Peter Whalley] (Harper & Row, 1963)

Space Age, Go Home (Ryerson Press, 1964)

100 Years of What? [with Peter Whalley] (Ryerson Press, 1966)

A Scar is Born (Ryerson Press, 1968)

Don't Move! (McClelland & Stewart, 1971)

Vancouver (Doubleday, 1970)

Still a Nicol (McGraw Hill Ryerson, 1972)

One Man's Media (Holt, Rinehart & Winston, 1973)

Letters to My Son (Macmillan, 1974)

Three Plays (Talonbooks, 1975)

There's A Lot of It Going Around (Doubleday, 1975)

Canada Cancelled Because of Lack of Interest
[with Peter Whalley] (Hurtig, 1977)

The Joy of Hockey [with David More] (Hurtig, 1978)

The Joy of Football [with David More] (Hurtig, 1980)

Golf — The Agony & the Ecstasy [with David More] (Hurtig, 1982)

Canadide (Macmillan, 1983)

Tennis — It Serves You Right (Hurtig, 1984)

How to . . . [with Graham Pilsworth] (Macmillan, 1985)

The U.S. or Us [with David More] (Hurtig, 1986)

Dickens of the Mounted (McClelland & Stewart, 1992)

Back Talk (McClelland & Stewart, 1992)

Skiing Is Believing [with David More] (Johnson Gorman Pub., 1995)

Anything for a Laugh (Harbour Pub., 1998)

When Nature Calls (Harbour Pub., 1999)

The
Casanova
Sexicon

*a manual
for liberated men*

⌁

Eric Nicol

RONSDALE PRESS

THE CASANOVA SEXICON
Copyright © 2001 Eric Nicol

RONSDALE PRESS
3350 West 21st Avenue
Vancouver, B.C., Canada
V6S 1G7

Set in New Baskerville: 11 pt on 15
Typesetting: Julie Cochrane
Printing: Hignell Printing, Winnipeg, Manitoba
Cover Design: Ewa Pluciennik
Author Photo: Barry Peterson & Blaise Enright-Peterson

Ronsdale Press wishes to thank the Canada Council for the Arts, the Government of Canada through the Book Publishing Industry Development Program (BPIDP), and the Province of British Columbia through the British Columbia Arts Council for their support of its publishing program.

NATIONAL LIBRARY OF CANADA CATALOGUING IN PUBLICATION DATA

Nicol, Eric, 1919–
    The Casanova sexicon

    ISBN 0-921870-88-4

    I. Men—Sexual behavior—Humor. 2. Casanova, Giacomo,
1725–1798—Humor. I. Title.
PS8527.I35C37 2001   C818'.5402   C2001-910602-5
PR9199.3.N5C37 2001

DEDICATED TO ALL
MY OLD GIRL FRIENDS —
AND WHY HAVEN'T YOU
ANSWERED MY LETTERS?

*"In love
with loving"*

— ST. AUGUSTINE (345-430)

a d v i s o r y

☙

This book may be unsuitable for
children under three years of age. Unless
accompanied by parents. Who have
bought the book, rather than borrowed or
shoplifted. Persons who have a physical
reaction to exposure to sexually explicit
material should read this book under
the care of a physician, or under the doctor
herself. The publisher is not legally
responsible for the views expressed by
Jacques Casanova *or* the author, and will
deny even having read the book.

The Time Was Ripe

Casanova *n* a man notorious for seducing women [G.J. Casanova de Seingalt. It. Adventurer d. 1798]

No man has ever brought immorality and immortality even closer together than they are in *The Concise Oxford Dictionary.*

Don Juan *n* a seducer of women; a libertine [name of a legendary Sp. nobleman celebrated in fiction, e.g. by Byron]

In the libertine derby, Don Juan loses out to Casanova. Mainly because he is fictional. In contrast, Giacomo was a fact of libidinous life. He wrote twelve volumes of memoirs, whereas Don Juan wrote nothing, not even a note for the milkman.

Also, Casanova was an Italian, Don Juan a Spaniard. Both peoples are warm-blooded, particularly in comparison to the English, who have produced no world-class seducer of women. But Italian lovers are less influenced by the bullfight than are Spaniards. Don Juan violated women, while Casanova delectated them. The Spanish letch used the ladies, the Italian cultivated their love. As American biographer Leonard Lewis Levinson so aptly observes: "Casanova was a Boy Scout who did his good deeds in bed."

If he had been a McCasanova, he could have boasted THOU-SANDS OF WOMEN SERVED.

Yet he never married. Today's man can only marvel at the sexual dexterity of this magician who could juggle dozens of belles in bed without once dropping his single status. What a role model!

How did Casanova manage to avoid nearly all the pitfalls of dalliance, with only an occasional stumble to remind him that coition with other than a virgin could bed him with the mother of all bugs?

Luckily, the man wrote a primer for the heterosexual male with a lively libido. Called it *The History of My Life*. His memoirs. In whose pages a disciple may find the keys to a rewarding sex life in the 21st century, as Casanova enjoyed it in the 18th.

The times are comparable, as a — dare we say? — hay day for the Lothario (who also shared Giacomo's century). Casanova's Europe was in a period of liberation — moral as well as intellectual — from the conventional.

In fashion, women were showing more bosom — a new horizon for the explorer in men.

Voltaire was letting the air out of Church dogma, and milking other sacred cows.

It was the period of the Enlightenment, and Casanova's mission was to enlighten women — as universally as possible — in his special area of expertise: sexology.

His was that era in continental Europe before the French Revolution came and ruined a perfectly corrupt society, by promoting high principles of democracy, that rather dull figment of imagination. The humbly born Casanova could still use the upscale bed as a trampoline, to vault up the social ladder, all the way to the king and, more influentially, to the king's mistress. He gained entrée to Madame de Pompadour herself, who distributed favours with a personal touch totally lost on Madame La Guillotine.

In France, and especially Paris, where Casanova foraged most successfully for *la femme*, the fashionable address was the Bastille. Everybody who was anybody was popped in there, with their servants, for being naughtier than the king. Louis XV himself never made it on the guest list. Too namby-pamby. When he died, the populace lined the route of his funeral to heckle "There goes The Ladies' Delight!" Their declaration stemmed from the common knowledge that his mistresses cheated on him, Madame du Barry in particular setting a new standard as the lay of the land.

But no lady was disloyal to Casanova, as the lover of choice. Although he complains in his memoirs that he has ever been "the dupe of women", they never took advantage of him, except financially, emotionally, socially, and spiritually. Sexually, he had their full attention. For as long as his stamina held up.

A Big Daddy, he wasn't.

To put it positively, Casanova was a heart specialist. He dedicated his life to researching the subtleties of the love affair. He had no other work to distract him from this career. He strove to be the professional who put the stud in studies.

Casanova was superbly equipped, mentally and physically, for the exploration of Love. Which to him presented the kind of challenge that Mount Everest held for Mallory. "Because it was there" was reason enough for him to conquer a woman's virtue, if she too was a beautiful, snowy-white eminence.

In another sense, Giacomo was a missionary whose god was Eros. His pilgrim's path ranged the length and breadth of Europe and even unto the Middle East, as he made converts to Priapism. His version of the missionary position was compatible with that of the Catholic Church. (True, Rome was not Casanova's favourite town. He much preferred the wild bayous of Venice, or Amsterdam, or Paris, over the Eternal City of the seven hills. He wasn't really into climbing.)

Yet Casanova was no moral kin to the characters of *Les Liaisons Dangereuses,* whose sport it was to aim the mind to wound the heart. Casanova didn't have a mean streak. If he broke a woman's heart it was an accident, usually covered by the insurance of her admission to a convent.

Nor did he lean towards the less subtle carnal romps recounted by the "Marquis" de Sade, who overdid the dissolution a tad in his novels. Nothing in the thousands of pages of his memoirs hints at S & M as part of Casanova's bag of erotic tricks, unless making love in a rocking carriage during a thunderstorm may be classified as sexual perversion.

However, the works of de Sade and de Laclos are an index of the maggoty morals from which Casanova profited so handsomely — with his gaming, his romantic intrigues, and display of his remarkable talent for conning the drawers off members of both genders.

As American humorist Will Cuppy observes in his hilarious essay, "Madame du Barry," her associates believed "we were put here to have a good time." Much the same philosophy, really, as that embraced by us folk boogeying into the new millennium. We have shucked off the mouldy-figism of the intervening Victorian period. If people feel the need of support from orthodox religion, they turn to their newspaper's Daily Horoscope, much as the 18th-century freethinkers doted on the numerology of which Casanova was a past master, spellbinding the full gamut of suckers.

The *grandes dames* that he met and mesmerized in France were the forerunners of today's career women. Clever, beautiful women have always managed to attain positions of wealth and power. The difference was that they could do it without having to get out of bed.

Casanova set the standard for respecting women's right to equal success. Contempt or disdain for the sex found no refuge in his spirit. He loved, or he didn't love. Sometimes he hated, but the victim was usually male. A Romeo with attitude, he wasn't. The oil with which he lubricated his seductions was refined not crude.

Casanova would have difficulty understanding the mean streak that plagues today's love affairs. Women's liberation has favored the contest of wills that complicates a relationship, to the detriment of simple lust. Instead of getting the hots for a woman, today's apprehensive swain has the luke-warms. And tepidity, however reasonable, does naught to enflame a woman's soul, let alone her body.

Yet the elemental, single-handed thrust of a Casanova's conquest is no less effective today, despite the painstaking analysis by women's magazines bent on putting the male's libido under the microscope, and dissecting a guy's motives with the clinical dispassion of a lab student examining the reproductive system of the frog.

Woman remains a female awaiting the ardent assault by the herd's dominant male. And Casanova was nothing if not the lord of the pride. He went everywhere with his trusty sword — which he used to bloody effect in several duels — plus a brace of pistols and a cane as back-up. A woman had merely to look at him to know, instantly, that she was in the presence of prize genes, ready to be transferred to her baby in a highly pleasurable process.

Thus Casanova's memoirs provide scripture and gospel for today's young man who wants to live a full sex life, totally uninhibited by a sense of spousal responsibility. Yet he may be reluctant to let the state take over all those functions — so restrictive to sexual promiscuity — that are now, for better or worse, assumed by daycare, social workers and a host of counsellors for the dysfunctional family. The rationale:

The man who pays his taxes has pretty well discharged his duty to society. To carry also the cross of being a support-paying, non-custodial, divorced male parent would be, to the Casanovan, a form of self-abuse.

To summarize, Jacques Casanova:

1. was a travelling salesman who carried his wares in his pants.
2. successfully resisted the urge to settle down, and the consequent need to settle up.
3. had no parental worries, only meeting his children socially.
4. lived a life free of mortgage payments, having no fixed address.

Casanova never had a steady job. Today's guy can relate to that situation, given that employment depends on the mobility to shift from position to position, as jobs appear and evanesce like the Cheshire Cat, with only a smile to replace the company pension.

At no time was doing an honest day's work part of Jacques' life game-plan, once he had realized that he was not really cut out to be a priest.

Casanova was all adaptor, no plug. His was an insecurity blanket, in which he wrapped himself and the pretty lady willing to share it.

In thus behaving as a non-domesticated animal, Casanova conformed to the mating habits of the males of most large mammal species: "Bam, bam, thank you, ma'am."

The species that mate for life are mostly birds. And not very bright birds, at that. Commitment lays an egg. If today's man yields to the pressure to model himself on the penguin, he can expect to spend a lot of time in a tux, and tend to walk funny.

Not our Casanova. Giacomo toured Europe as the prototypical male marking his territory. He used the same part of his anatomy as the wolf, ranging the Continent to claim women, with even a brief emission in London.

House-husband material, Casanova definitely was not. We find no mention in his exhaustive memoirs of his ever having had to cook a meal for himself, let alone for a date. He always had a chef, however makeshift, and a server. Even when jailed in The Leads, the Venice Inquisition hoosegow, Casanova contrived to get Room Service from the guard.

Everything he writes about his dining habits indicates that having to peel a potato would have made him impotent.

No meal was so delicious, for this adventurer *par excellence,* as that which he shared with a comely girl: gustatory prelude to making love. Time and again, he demonstrated that the Italian touch was more than ordering in a pizza. Casanova *wooed* women into bed, via the buffet. Sometimes in a matter of minutes, other times not till after dessert.

Besides being a gracious host, Jacques was a practising poet, who used his talent for verse-making to put his ardour in writing. Today's suitor thinks he can get the same effect by just turning up the volume on his stereo. Not likely.

Casanova understood, and no man better, that the attention given is returned two-fold in the pleasure gained. Seduction is sedulous.

Yes, Mr. Ever Ready was a gentleman, verbally at least. His memoirs' accounts of lively seduction, though graphic, never lapse into vulgar parlance. He is able to describe the most outrageous scenes without once using a word that would offend Mrs. Grundy, or even Mr. Grundy. He lends charm to a body function which, viewed by a non-participant, is not the stuff of classical ballet.

Shakespeare's "beast with two backs" is not heard grunting with exertion. One or two translators of *The History of My Life* into English (from the French) have tried to embellish, or rather debellish, Casanova's lyrical sex scenes with more earthy prose. These have been dismissed as counterfeit porn.

Today, "talking dirty" has its school of acolytes, as the most effective way to charm a woman. The bar-stool invocation — "Wanna fuck?" — may enchant some women, but likely they are already in an advanced state of alcoholic rapture.

Casanova has occasional resort to the instant relief afforded by such sluts, at the cost of sexually transmitted disease. But most of his campaigns called for all his resources of suasion, verbal as well as physical. He may have been Mother Nature's fool, expending much time and money, energy and talent, just to comply with the reproductive imperative of all species. But he did make it a class act.

Had he enjoyed the facility of e-mail, Jacques Casanova might have cut such a swath through the womanhood of the world that all other men would curse Bill Gates and the microchip that made him.

Was Casanova *always* a gentleman, in satisfying his gargantuan sexual appetite? Well, no. He was the first to admit that fair play was not inevitably part of his game plan. He was perfectly candid about his ethical values. "I don't have any," he said. And, being free of these impediments himself, he resented being confronted by them in women he fancied.

Casanova firmly believed that love conquers all — including moral scruples. Women who used these anchors to prevent their being swept away by his surging passion infuriated him. He saw it as abnormal, a crime against nature, for a woman not to "love" as physically as he was prepared to "love." Against their resistance he had no qualms about employing any means short of violence, to have his way with them.

What is extraordinary is that he recounts such unflattering episodes with complete honesty, knowing that his behaviour was reprehensible. He damns himself, to demonstrate the inexorable power of his desire. A compulsion that women found exciting.

Faint heart never won fair, lady.

The man who shows undue respect for a woman's virtue is insulting her attractiveness. (La Rochefoucauld: "What we see as strength of will may be only weakness of desire.")

Every woman yearns to be ravished; none to be raped.

So, if necessary, Casanova erred on the side of force, rather than affront the lady by displaying feeble purpose. Just as the breaking of eggs is requisite to the making of the omelette, the making of madame may require more than preserving her shell of maidenly modesty.

Yes, Casanova was, at times, a cad. A real rotter. His strong-arm tactics do not commend themselves to our Casanovan unless he really relishes the prospect of making car licence plates in somewhat spartan quarters. Luckily, virtue is not as vital to the prosperity of our liberated woman, making token resistance expendable.

But discussion of Casanova's sexual expertise can over-shadow the fact that this was a man of many parts, not all of them below the waist. He could have become very successful in many another line of endeavour — finance, clergy, diplomatic service, music (he played the fiddle), and professional gambling. He wrote like an angel, but — until he sat down as an old man to write his memoirs — his main readers were the enchanted women to whom his private letters showed that ink can be the ultimate love potion.

Ergo, in our time as in Casanova's, the formula for his success with women will not suffice for today's disciple unless he has the wit fit to woo. Almost any man willing to learn, however, must profit from close attention to the living text of the memoirs, pausing only to close the mouth agape at the mastery demonstrated by this copulative genius.

To repeat: the alphabetical excerpts that follow cannot be as fulfilling as reading the complete *The History of My Life,* a work of over a million words. But the reader is not getting any younger. And, young or old, a man should find in these pages enlightenment, and treatment for why he is watching too much sport on television to assure survival of our species.

Take one letter a day, of the insights of the world's greatest lover.

☙ Abode

Where to live? The first question that the budding Casanovan should consider, but rarely does. There is just one place where he wants to be able to hang his hat, and that's obscene.

Having a permanent address is simply not in the cards. Giacomo never had one [*see* NOMADISM], man or boy, and none of the scores of women with whom he mated persuaded him — if indeed they even tried — to help her build a nest.

Casanova sensed, instinctively, that having a mortgage could cause erectile dysfunction.

Nor did owning his own home attract him as a goal worth working towards. The only part of a house that held any lasting attraction for him was the bedroom. If the bedroom had an en-suite bathroom, with a spacious tub, that was a plus, but other rooms were optional.

That his women and his servants spent time in these supplementary chambers was something he understood to be necessary, so long as it wasn't overdone.

Some men find comfort in sleeping in their own bed. Casanova avoided this situation as much as possible.

He tested more mattresses than Sealy.

Also his memoirs record no instance of his having to make his own bed — a repulsive undertaking. That function, and others, fell to hotel maids, hosts' wives and manservants who were too scared of the boss to question their job description.

Some potential Casanovans, especially those still in college taking courses other than those on the campus restaurant menu, are still living at home with their parents, being too strapped financially to afford their own flat. A real drawback, this can be, to free-wheeling womanizing. When Mom is still doing your laundry, you have to be inordinately nervous about strange stains on underwear . . . a safe stuck in your sock . . . a savagely ripped shirt . . .

No, his calling requires the Casanovan to be footloose and fancy free, a pilgrim setting forth from the missionary position.

A rolling stone gathers no missis.

➣ Abracadabra

As a sorcerer, Giacomo Casanova was a Harry Potter with a sharper focus.

His being impressed with the power of hocus-pocus happened when he was only six years old. Up to that time the boy — both of whose parents had buzzed off as travelling players — had been mute. A dubious asset in a future lover. He also suffered from fierce nocturnal nosebleeds, another drawback in the sexual embrace.

Then his medical case is taken over by a local witch — presumably a referral from the old priest who was Jacques' guardian. Her cure: to bathe his body with exotic oils and shut him up in a box, while chanting spells and incantations even weirder than what we now hear from our personal psychotherapist.

While boxed, little Jacques has a vision of a beautiful female spirit, who kisses him and vanishes.

Presto! The lad emerges from the box talking a blue streak. Nosebleeds, nil. More miraculous yet, Casanova learns to read, in the national record time of one month. (A tempting example for today's parent, casting about for a tutor to help Junior with his English. But because of our starchy remedial-education standards, oiling and crating a child does not compute.)

So it was that magical transformations were second nature to Casanova, later in life. Notably with the laying on of hands that turned dumbstruck virgins into women of the world. Or at least of their neighborhood.

~ Abracadabra 2

First, however, it was a teenage Giacomo who profited from the experience of magical ministration to the ailing. He was scraping by, literally, as second fiddle in a no-name band, the night he happened to be sharing a taxi gondola with an elderly and rich senator, when the latter suffered a stroke. The lad assisted the senator home and stayed at his bedside for days, while various doctors came and went, their prescriptions ineffectual. When the senator at last recovered, he was so grateful for Casanova's curative presence that he virtually adopted the kid. Gave him money. Introduced him to Venetian society. And thus the young man got the credentials he needed to become a professional spellbinder.

His most notable, and profitable, patient that he was later to enjoy: the spectacularly spaced-out Parisian plutocrat, Madame d'Urfé. Casanova ministered mightily to this elderly fruitcake's manic wish to have her spirit transmitted into the body of a male infant, so that she might begin a new life as a horny young hunk. The deluxe make-over.

Spiritual transmutation, with a side order of sex? No problem for her consummate care-provider. Casanova prescribed a lengthy program of exercises that would need substantial financing. (None of his services qualified for Medicare.)

It was many years before Mme d'Urfé twigged to the fact that her being effed (once) by her practitioner had not yielded the kind of return she expected from her investment.

The episode that raised her hopes more readily than it did Casanova's penis stands as one of the classics of situation comedy. Unable to become aroused by the sight of the waiting recumbent crone, he is obliged to hire a whore to wait in an adjoining chamber, dash in to get pumped, and rush back to perform the most demanding intrusive procedure of his career. He was not Johns Hopkins, but the man did have moxie.

May the Casanovan profit from this example of psychic broker-age, now that wealthy beldams can take a dip in the sperm pool? Probably not. [*See* OLDER WOMEN] Metaphysiotherapy could become trendy again, but at present may not be worth your buying the stethoscope.

☞ Adoration

"I enjoyed her adoration," writes Casanova of Rosalie, "this enticing fifteen-year-old beauty. Her charms left nothing to be desired . . . 'You shall be my mistress,' I said, 'and my servants shall respect you as if you were my wife.'"

Clearly, *adoration* can be heady stuff. What Casanova promised Rosalie was as close to marriage as he was apt to venture, while sober.

Today, it is harder for the Casanovan to win a girl's adoration, even at fifteen, because females are too likely to be well informed — by the accursed media, movies and Oprah — that men are flawed beings at best.

Under scrutiny, a young woman's adoration of a man usually proves to be INFATUATION. Which, of course, is a Bad Thing. Infatuation can quickly degrade into hatred, which can result in a man's being hauled into court charged with sexual assault, stalking, molestation, and ecological damage to the habitat of the cross-eyed hoot owl.

In the worst-case scenario, he has a valued appendage lopped off while he slumbers, by a woman who has experienced a sharp drop-off in devotion.

Also, the specifics for being adored by a woman are elusive. Otherwise *every* man would be being adored by a woman, and statistics indicate that female adoration of men is not only less than 100 percent but not as prevalent as, say, herpes. And there may be a connection between those stats.

What about the man who contracts adoration of a woman? This can easily happen, as men are more romantic than women. (Who but men have written the romantic love songs, before the genre was taken over by dirges moaned by female icons of angst?)

The drinking bars of the western world are festooned with guys who have loved not wisely but too well. Or who trudge our myriad fairways, in that crazed surrogate intercourse whose goal is to penetrate a small orifice less challenging than that of the girl they teed up on a pedestal.

Only *the* Casanova could successfully adore all women. It was what he did instead of walking on water.

⊸ Adultery

Harder to define, today. (If a married female feminist has sexual relations with a single heterosexual man, is it adultery or bestiality?)

Casanova lived in a less ambiguous moral climate. He cuckolded more husbands — and still stayed alive — than probably any other adulterer of record. The old Test's injunction against the venereal sin was not the first thing that came to his mind when he encountered a pretty woman who just happened to be some other guy's wife. And such were his powers of seduction that even the most Commandments-respecting woman was obliged to put No. 7 on hold.

Yet Casanova was not one of those men — pitiful creatures — who persuade a wife to cheat on her husband because the seduction bolsters their self-esteem. This happens often in business offices. Instance: the well-known Canadian newspaper columnist, who tolerated his paltry pay with the help of cheap scotch, and whose revenge consisted of his banging the publisher's wife, in the publisher's office, and *on the publisher's desk*. Wrong motivation.

Casanova, however, was never moved to commit adultery by anything but pure lust. On one notable occasion, he scored the double: "a beautiful Roman named Lucrezia" married to a lawyer, "Franceso Castelli, a pleasant middle-aged man," both accompanied by her sister Angelique, whose obliging fiancé, Don Francisco, invites them all to overnight at his villa.

Casanova takes full advantage of the circumstance that Lucrezia has contrived to bed down with her sister in a room handy to that of the eternal opportunist . . .

"What ecstasies of love from the very onset! What delicious raptures succeeded each other! . . . " Having rogered the lawyer's wife to a fair-thee-well, and deflowered the sister affianced to their host, Casanova enjoys the morning-after call of the antlered advocate:

"He was reproaching them for sleeping too long. Then knocking at my door, he threatened to bring the ladies to me if I didn't get out of bed!"

The girls' rosy cheeks and smiling eyes at the ensuing breakfast capped yet another of Casanova's triumphs in human relations (everybody happy) that make us marvel at the man's prodigious talent for overcoming propriety.

However, in this matter of adultery, Giacomo may not provide a viable role model for today's liberated man. For one thing, lawyers are not as trusting as they appear to have been in Casanova's time. And sisters seem less willing to share a source of pleasure, sibling rivalry having become a recognized factor in the dysfunctional family.

Also, Casanova had a unique ability — possibly impossible to duplicate — to put the horns on hubbies who were almost grateful to have their wives transformed into radiantly happy women. The make-over might not be permanent, but by the time it wore off, Casanova would have skipped town.

Conclusion: for the Casanovan, committing adultery presumes your leaving no forwarding address.

⮑ Advances

Sexual advances on women fall into two (2) categories:

   (A) Wanted

   (B) Unwanted

By his own account, Casanova scored almost 100% class A advances. Every time he stepped up to the plate — usually the dinner plate of a cozy dinner for two — he hit a home run. He rarely, if ever, struck out, even though he might have had to foul off a few pitches for commitment.

What is the determining factor in the success of a man's sexual advance? Aside, that is, from whether the advancer has the build of a gnome and the personality of a gargoyle?

The determinant is, does his advance reflect:

1. self-confidence, or
2. smug assumption, or
3. plain ineptitude?

Casanova, of course radiated number 1. The more women he seduced (starting early in life), the less reason he had to suspect that he would be other than warmly welcomed into the arms, and other regions, of the woman he had in his sights.

Yet he never allowed this self-confidence to degrade to number 2, the taking for granted that he was God's gift to the entire female sex. To Casanova, every beautiful woman was a new and fascinating land to be explored. And, sometimes, populated. She had but to look into his eyes, to read the high sperm count. Without presumption, he epitomized the Life Force that Bernard Shaw dissipated in writing until he was too old to do much else.

But it is determinant number 3 that the Casanovan — sensitive and untried creature that he is — may represent in his advances to women. While shyness is much less off-putting to a woman than his being grossly cocky, today's woman is usually too busy to interpret blushing diffidence. She may just assume that the applicant is (a) gay, (b) transsexual, or (c) undecided.

Bashful, Casanova wasn't. He had the Italian male's natural talent for making physical contact with a woman from the get-go of meeting — the reason why so many British and North American women book onto tours of the Mediterranean.

An Italian train porter can do more in helping a female tourist to board her carriage than she has had from her husband since the honeymoon.

Therefore the Casanovan must go boldly forth into the space of a woman's attention. Don't wait for the lady to drop her handkerchief. Most women carry Kleenex, these days, and are schooled not to litter.

And he must be open to a woman's advances. If the gorgeous girl you've just met asks you for your phone number, don't assume that she is a realtor. Other women wear high heels too. Think positive and invest in Cupid's hardware: an answering machine.

∼ Advantages

As in other fields of accomplishment, it starts with the genes.

Casanova was born with creative talent. A glance at our standard encyclopedia reveals the genetic factor: a cluster of glittering Casanovas: the brothers Giovanni Batista Casanova and Francesco Guiseppe Casanova, both painters whose works achieved international notice, despite their scattered upbringing from the shambles of a family.

The seed assured the success of the family.

Giacomo most famously displayed his artistry not on canvas but on the mattress. Like his brothers he had multiple talents which, had he not been dilettante, could have won him lasting fame as a poet, or playwright, or mathematician, or historian, or any one of a dozen other genres of genius. But he chose to focus most of his natural skills on the wooing of beautiful women. And who's to say that he had it wrong?

For the Casanovan, the message is that one's deriving from a good, stable home — teething on the silver spoon — is not requisite for success as a great lover. Giacomo's early life was chaos: father dead, mother an itinerant dancer; dependence on Grandma and some weird clergy. But his spirit of enquiry regarding natural phenomena — namely girls — was indomitable. It saved him from an obscure career in the priesthood, where his God-given gift for SEDUCTION would have had to struggle to survive.

Nor did he profit from having the romantic profile of a Valentino. Mouth too mini. Rather weak chin. Nose too largely Roman.

Hair not naturally wavy. Only Casanova's eyes were prepossessing, compelling a woman's attention to the below-the-neck attributes that gave women a rush, more or less directly to the bed.

Early on he understood that the wisest use of money is to spend it on women. Women nearly always provide a generous return on a man's investment. And the interest they pay creates the most pleasurable form of inflation.

Conclusion: the would-be Casanovan who, for a date, is ashamed to borrow his parents' aging car because the stereo lacks decibels, will never attain the status of our revered Venetian.

To be given a healthy body and lively mind is all the endowment fund one needs.

~ Ambiance

Casanova understood the importance of a romantic setting, for seducing a nun. Or, indeed, any woman with whom an assignation has been laid on. He could perform well in the impromptu situation — a gondola, a carriage, a bit of shrubbery — but to ensure a prolonged and inimitable night of amatory delight he took the trouble to create an atmosphere that would not take No for an answer.

Casanova could, indeed, have given lessons to *Playboy* publisher Hugh Hefner, despite the motorized, planetary bed.

His attention to ambiance was typically Italian, as anyone knows who has examined the bedroom murals of homes in the ruined Pompeii. (Where the original vibrating bed was enjoyed, though briefly.)

Here, for instance, is Casanova's account of the logistics of his preparation for the invasion of Sister Marie-Madeleine:

. . . I rented a casino which suited my purpose exactly. It had belonged to the last English ambassador and I had it for a hundred sequins until Easter. It consisted of five rooms furnished in the most elegant style, and everything was arranged

for love, pleasure and good cheer. The service of the dining-
room was made through a sham window in the wall, provided
with a dumb-waiter revolving upon itself, and fitting the window so exactly that masters and servants could not see each
other. The décor of the apartment was magnificent. There
was an octagonal room, the walls, the ceiling and the floor of
which were entirely covered with splendid Venetian mirrors,
arranged in such a manner as to reflect on all sides every
position of the amorous couple enjoying the pleasures of love.
The walls of the drawing-room were covered with small squares
of real china, representing little cupids and naked amorous
couples in all sorts of attitudes, well calculated to excite the
imagination. Elegant and very comfortable sofas were placed
on convenient corners. There was a bath in Carrara marble
and a clock with an alarm which could be set at any hour . . .

Quite a leap from renting Unit 6 of the Junction Motel. Venetian
blinds notwithstanding.

Today's Casanova is apt to flatter himself that his apartment will
serve as an effective trysting place so long as he turns on the stereo
and orders in a medium pizza.

Yet it takes more than removal of dirty laundry from the coffee-
table to convince a lady that this is other than a service call.

So, did Casanova get a good return on his rental of an ambassador's casino? It was, indeed, a lease on life, a sex life such as blesses
few men except in their more erotic dreams. The episode stands as
a lesson to today's man, who too often expects his date to provide
the apartment, the home-made gourmet dinner, and the sex on the
floor, all as a package deal paid for with the inevitable bottle of
Bolivian wine.

Attention to detail. We need it as much to fashion a memorable
relationship as to caulk our sailboat or wax our skis. Our mating
dance should be at least as elaborate as that of the prairie chicken.

In love, as in other of life's enterprises, we get what we pay for.

ᨓ Amusement

"I had a great talent for making others laugh while I kept a serious countenance myself. I had learnt that accomplishment from M. de Malipiero, my first master in the art of good breeding, who used to say to me:

"If you wish your audience to cry, you must shed tears yourself, but if you wish to make them laugh, you must continue to look serious as a judge."

Facially animated in passion, but solemn to make the lady laugh: Casanova knew the formula for amusing madame. And the importance of evoking a woman's laughter, as part of beguiling her, cannot be overestimated.

Women love to laugh. Some analysts of the most effective factors in a man's attractiveness to a woman give top place to his ability to draw a giggle. This talent requires something more subtle than placement of a whoopee cushion. Or off-colour jokes. Or the ability to fold one's lower lip over one's nose.

Tickling a woman's fancy is not a manual exercise. It is a verbal skill. Wherein lies the deadpan delivery known to every great comedian, from Chaplin to Fields to Keaton to Woody Allen. The last of these has had incredible success in captivating beautiful women half his age, despite his having the physique and features of a somewhat haggard gnome.

How? By making them laugh. An extremely intelligent individual, Allen has used his acute awareness of his inadequacies as a springboard for the wry observations that women find more entertaining than smugly smiling good looks.

Casanova appears to have ben blessed with the same acute sense that life is a farce that must be played straight. He honoured women with not only the total commitment of his commanding body but also the dry wit that kept them titillated between the orgasmic groans.

Giacomo displayed precociousness as a wit, the story being told that, at age twelve, he attended a waggish dinner where the question was raised: why in Latin grammar is the word for vagina a masculine noun, while the word for penis is a feminine noun? The lad's sally: "Because the servant takes its name from the master."

Adept with the one-liner or not, the Casanovan should keep in mind that a woman is won by his lips long before his meet hers.

The smile is consummated with the kiss.

ᕼ Andromania

"At the Church of the Good Success I saw the Duchess of Villadorias, notorious for her andromania. When the *furor uterinus* seized her, nothing could keep her back. She would rush at the man who had excited her and he had no choice but to satisfy her passion. This had happened several times in public assemblies and had given rise to some extraordinary scenes, yet she was still both young and pretty."

Probably every Casanovan fantasizes at times about being sexually assaulted by a Duchess of Villadorias, though perhaps not at a hockey game or other public event where he is holding a hot-dog.

Andromania and its lusty sister, nymphomania, still exist as sexual phenomena, though they always seem to be something that happens to some other guy. Only in his dreams does the Casanovan get ravished by a gorgeous, implacable and insatiable virago who also offers to pay for his ripped shirt and ravaged shorts.

Casanova himself does not report having been attacked by any andromaniacs, which suggests that the philanderer is not the prey of choice for this species of woman. She is more likely to target the shy and unsuspecting. Yes, that young, good-looking kid who has gone to the seminar on retirement financial planning with nothing on his mind but government bonds and other safe investments.

How should the Casanovan deal with a beautiful and wealthy woman who seizes the initiative — and God knows what else — in her pathological sexual frenzy? Is he taking advantage of a sick mind if he yields to her demand for immediate satisfaction, in the elevator or other spartan milieu?

Well, again, Hell hath no fury, etc. Sometimes it is necessary to sublimate our ethical misgivings in the interest of gender equality. Women have every right to come on to a man vigorously. It may not conform to the mating pattern of other mammals, such as lions and moose. But everything in nature evolves. The Casanovan may simply be caught up in the wave of the future. Be ready to surf.

☞ Anecdotes

Casanova dined out on his stories. Reciprocally, the anecdotes with which he delectated social gatherings opened the door to more adventures. And — O, facts can be so cruel! — women are attracted to a man who is popular.

Thus, in his mouth Casanova had the generator of a lively life.

Did he — as is sometimes said of today's sexually graphic novelists — live it up so that he could write it down? If so, he waited a very long time to cash in, with his memoirs. More evident is that it was verbally that he charmed company, and especially the female component.

Jacques' story of his escape from The Leads prison, for example, won him a place at the finest dinner tables in France and elsewhere that *le haut monde* gathered to gape with admiration. Did he embellish the facts of that incredible exit from the Inquisition's prize pokey? Probably. Who cared? Maybe he just walked out while a guard was momentarily blinded by a bribe. No matter. The tale, as told by the handsome, dashing rake, was a godsend to any hostess, and one that made the ladies present bite their napkins in the first spasm of lust.

You, the Casanova disciple, will therefore enhance your image as a daring adventurer if:

(a) you have travelled, farther than the local A&W.

(b) when you tell the mixed guests that you have just returned from Aspen or Whistler, you have actually skied there.

(c) you are widely believed to have escaped custody, in some country that does not have extradition rights in your hostel.

Yes, being a magnetic raconteur makes special demands, especially if speaking in company makes you incontinent. Start small, at a table with male chums in a sport bar, and work your way up to a night course in welding.

The stories we write may win us admiration, but it's the yarns we tell that get us loved.

⇜ Aphrodisiacs

"We dined and amused one another, in the voluptuous fashion of lovers, sucking oysters off the tongue of each other. Passionate reader, try it, and tell me that it is not the gods' own nectar!"

Another reason, here, why taking one's date to eat at a Wendy's may not hack it, for the wannabe Casanovan. Even in the more expensive restaurants, slurping oysters tongue-to-tongue will draw the attention of the head-waiter, as well as chilling stares from other diners concerned about endangered species of shellfish.

Casanova took care to produce his divine nectar in the private dining-room, adjoining a boudoir whose library specialized in erotic illustrations: ". . . whose enflaming style obliges the reader to seek the reality of the image they presented." The Casanovan who leaves around a copy of *The Reader's Digest,* to impress his guest with his intellectual interests, is sending a mixed message at a time when clarity of purpose is essential.

"A book at bedtime" had special meaning for Casanova. Although denied the instructive images of photography and video, he made the most of old engravings that fanned the flame of passion without being downright Kama Sutran.

They put the tit in titillation.

Casanova also burned a lot of incense at the altar of Love. Thus he enlisted all five senses for the sortie against a woman's virtue. If she didn't have any virtue, he could reduce the overhead. But when the defended hill had to be taken, he spared no expense to assure victory.

His WINE bill alone, for instance, would have beggared someone less lucky at the gaming table. He speaks of the heavy casualties, as many as twenty bottles of champagne in a single engagement. How many of his disciples are prepared to sacrifice more than a single bottle of Okanagan Red?

Should the Casanovan heed the current medical research that suggests that consuming alcohol actually impairs the libido? Well, perhaps the experiments hold true for mice, but it is hard to get a giggle out of rodents even when they're sober.

However, he would never have resorted to something like knock-out drops in a drink, to which some desperate oafs resort today. Necrophilia held no attraction for Casanova. On the contrary, his lady's token resistance, despite the aphrodisiacs, served to intensify his ardour, and the visible/audible evidence of her intense pleasure was vital to the ensemble climax.

The sure thing is less fun.

～ Appliances

Visiting England, home of the nascent Industrial Revolution, Casanova had one of his few contacts with mechanical aids to sex. He was approached at his lodging by a salesman lugging an armchair, for which he was asking 100 guineas. He demonstrated the hi-tech seating, which had five springs:

"They come into play all the same time, when anyone sits down. Two springs seize the two arms and hold them tightly, while two others separate the legs, and the fifth raises the seat."

When the vendor sat in this charming armchair, the hope that springs eternal forced him into the posture of a woman in the labor room. "And your business is done."

Only in England, you say.

Casanova was momentarily tempted to buy the *chaise d'amour,* in the end denying Progress because "it might easily have sent me to the gallows." Whose sprung trap-door would have cost him dearly indeed.

Casanova appears to have had little need of sex appliances like the restraining armchair. He travelled light, as a rule. Today he might have developed a dependence on the motel's vibrating bed, or other jiggling that lacks conversation. He would be more aware of the romantic potential of handcuffs that promise a permanent relationship with a bed-post. *Plus ça change . . .*

Perhaps because his first lovers were nuns, none of whom carried a whip, chains or a pool table, Casanova seems to have ignored the concept of the dominatrix. He never mentions getting spanked, a Tory member of Britain's parliament not being one of his several personae.

Indeed, Casanova's memoirs serve as a challenge to the lovers of our time to rely less on sex toys that they were not born with. When Casanova finally became impotent, it was not because the batteries died. He had a built-in generator of love's juice. Fueled only by the solar power of a woman's smile.

～ Architecture

"Certainly, I am a good architect, and I think you're magnificently built."

Casanova was responding to a question from a young lady with whom he was in bed, along with her sister, who had whipped off the covers to reveal her sister naked.

"Are you satisfied with me?"

When Casanova tries to corroborate his first impression, she demurs: "Stay, my dear. Don't touch me. It's enough that you have seen me."

Casanova the architect is quick to explain the limitations of visual impression: "Alas, it is by touching that one rectifies the mistakes of the eyes. One judges by smoothness and firmness. Let me kiss those two fair sources of life. I esteem them more than the hundred breasts of Cybele."

Although he had ample opportunity to study the architecture of other domed wonders in the great cities of Europe — St. Paul's Cathedral comes to mind — his memoirs are devoid of special attention. It is with the tight focus of his particular discipline that Casanova concentrates on the specifics of the perfect feminine form. When he speaks — as he often does — of the "temple of Love," he is referring to the *mons veneris* where he worshipped daily, weather permitting.

(In his building-inspection of women's pectoral balcony, Casanova was spared today's hazard of admiring as natural cleavage what is in fact a silicon valley. Renovation lurks everywhere.)

While he also took an interest in the design of a woman's face, her torso was the area of his architectural expertise. He was not a leg man. The ladies' dress fashion of the era concealed the limbs but exposed a lot of BREASTS. Yet Casanova did not rush to judgment. Not till the corset was safely dismantled, and the wearer "in a state of nature," did he ardently confirm his first impression.

That favorable impression could, however, be compromised by the woman's FEET. Big feet negated a big bosom, in his esteem, proving the importance of the unobtrusive substructure.

⤳ Arousal

Hard it is, to say which can be the more embarrassing:

    (A) erectile dysfunction, or
    (B) erectile overfunction

Problem A has received a lot of attention, since drugs like Viagra goosed the market into a massive response. But Problem B — inadvertent erection, in an inappropriate setting (dance floor, hospital bed, funeral service, etc.) — is a gaffe in the sight of man and God.

Casanova recounts such an accident. Incurred in his salad days: at an elegant garden party he meets a lovely young thing who excites him — it is a warm day, and he is wearing linen breeches that show the lust — when she examines his watch-fob. Manually. Result:

". . . a natural but involuntary excitement caused me to be very indiscreet."

The lady pretends to be "vexed," and he is left feeling deep shame, as well as too tight in the crotch. The old memoirist reflects:

"Such was my delicacy of feeling in those days. I used to credit people with exalted sentiments, which often existed only in my imagination. I must confess that time has entirely destroyed that delicacy . . ."

Indeed. Today countless young men — Casanovans in the bud — suffer the same mortification of being visibly aroused in the presence of a woman. Who of course would never admit that she is inviting that response by fondling their watch-fob.

The Casanovan should keep in mind that women — superb realists that they are — recognize a man's sexual arousal as the most sincere compliment that they can hope to receive.

To validate his inspecting gaze, there is nothing more convincing than the involuntary salute.

Also, the chance of his creating offence has been reduced by today's badinage: "Is that a banana in your pocket or are you just glad to see me?"

If the Casanovan is really concerned about his hair-trigger arousal, however, and especially if a video camera is recording the event, he may elect to wear tights, as do male film actors faced with a torrid love scene. The baseball catcher's cup is another option, if you don't mind complicating a visit to the men's washroom.

～ Artistry

Other artists have worked in oils, or marble, or music, or driftwood garnished with bottle caps. Casanova the artist worked in love. His chosen medium was sex exalted into the supreme sentiment.

His transient masterpiece: Lady in Ecstasy.

Like the clay sculptor, Casanova worked with his hands, to create love. And masterful was his hand in the drawing of a sigh.

Like the glassblower, he used his lips to fashion the finished *objet d'art*. Love.

And like the composer — for in fact Casanova preluded his career with playing the violin — he employed his voice (a sexophone?) as music that hath charms to soothe the savage breast.

Such artistic talent came naturally to this Italian born to the visible heritage of the birthplace of the Renaissance. What he accomplished with love suggests what Michelangelo might have done had he been heterosexual.

Casanova had to create his love works without the patronage of a pope. He was subsidized only by Lady Luck, with whom he had a lifelong affair.

Alas, Casanova's was an artwork that died with him. What he produced in love lived on only in the innumerable love babies he created. Bonny bastards. His genes no doubt survive, probably thrive, in countless persons world-wide, most of them unaware that they owe their artistic flair to love's non-resident genius, the man who gave them everything distinguishing, except his name.

Such is the pity, that his works were unsigned, and that for Paris the Eiffel Tower is the more remembered erection.

Assignation

"A secret meeting, especially between illicit lovers" — *The Concise Oxford Dictionary.*

In his sexual education, Casanova majored in Assignation. He had a natural flair for the subject, happily repeating the experiments to prove that stolen sweets *are* best, and fattening only to the female if she's not careful.

Typical is his assignation with the attractive wife of the Mayor of Cologne, the lady being so taken with him on short acquaintance as to show him how, by hiding in the church adjoining the Mayor's house, Casanova can wait till the beadle closes up for the night, then nip up a secret staircase that will gain him admission — and much more — to the wife's bedchamber. Her written instructions include the warning: ". . . there must be no spitting, coughing or nose-blowing. It would be fatal."

This element of risk-taking — extreme sport, if you like — is pure catnip, to Casanova. The excitement of intercourse during which nose-blowing can cost you your life: this is sex lived on the edge.

"The second night was delicious, but not so much as the former, since the Mayor was just beyond the partition. We could not see each other, and the violence of our ecstatic combats was restrained in his presence . . ."

Well, probably no assignation is perfect. The thrill of the forbidden fruit is sometimes flawed by the pits.

For Casanova, the assignation was spiced up by his having it off with the wife, daughter, mother, mistress, courtesan or female staff of an eminence, from a mayor to a reigning monarch of Europe. But he was not one to flaunt his success. A man of less principle would likely blab about his hanging the horns on the mighty, like the guy from the gas company telling his pub mates how he lit the pilot light for the chatelaine of a west-side mansion. Casanova was discreet, till he told all — nearly all — much later in his memoirs.

In our time, the assignation is apt to be a rather tawdry tryst between a married person of either sex and a lover, in a motel or hotel room richly furnished with guilt. Hardly anyone hides in a church these days, though as noted by Casanova, the Devil has more power in church than anywhere else.

Should the Casanovan eschew the assignation, as a game not worth the church candle? Probably. "Illicit lovers" has such a quaint ring in this time of sexual libertarianism that the experience has become *vieux chapeau*.

Besides, a person can still be legally sued for alienation of affection — a potential killer of your after-glow.

☞ Attention

Casanova never had a problem with gaining a woman's attention. His animal magnetism was strong enough to draw iron filings, let alone a female creature of flesh and blood.

He cut a figure to make the Sphinx herself blink, and his gaze performed laser surgery on any woman's moral scruples.

He had no need to push himself upon his willing prey. He understood The First Law of Attention Dynamics: the curiosity of the most beautiful woman in the room increases in ratio to the man's ignoring her . . . initially. By making a point of talking to the homeliest, unattended guest on the premises, the gentleman not only earns brownie points for social grace but also piques the belle's desire to see whether he has frontal features to complement his great buns.

At no time in his career did Casanova feel required to put a Personals ad in the Venice *Herald:*

"Mature SWM connoisseur of casinos wishes to meet S or M young virgin F who enjoys sex in a gondola . . ."

Casanova received ample, unsolicited attention from A-grade women at formal dinners, balls, the theatre and the carnivals where his roguish regard shone right through the black harlequin mask. It is fair to say that these settings were more romantic than today's rock concert or rave. (Some men may benefit from being unable to make themselves heard, but they are not true Casanovans.)

Casanova knew that getting a woman's attention, without firing a flare, was only half the battle of winning the rest of her:

"As to failure, I confess I did not give it a moment's thought, for there is not a woman in the world who can resist constant and loving attentions, especially when her lover is ready to make great sacrifices."

Message: picking up the tab at McDonald's is but a start in the vital role of paying attention to a woman. "Casual" may serve to describe sex, but love has a higher price tag.

☞ Attitude

Don Juan was the womanizer with an attitude. Giacomo Casanova did not carry one.

It's an important distinction, for the apprentice who should check *his* motivation, as conscientiously as he does his socks — for bad smell.

That ill odour distinguishes the difference between the two classic masters of seducing women. Many commentators have made a meal of the comparison of "these two primal forms of eroticism" (Stefan Zweig, *Casanova*). All agree: Jacques was the more lovable lecher; Don Giovanni, the nobler born, the likelier to go heel-kicking down to Hell. For humping ladies without respecting them.

Some warning signs, Casanovan:

1. You are taking up women to compensate for your failing to make the football team.

2. You are snobbish about the women you choose to seduce. You shun the shop girl, even though she fondles your credit card, in favour of the lady of high station. So that she has farther to fall from grace. You are into the Spanish John.

   (Casanova, however, was as happy bedding a chambermaid as a king's mistress. His was one of the more exemplary forms of democracy.)

3. You get your major jollies from debauching virgins. For Casanova, the making of a maiden was never a major breakthrough. He reports [*see* VIRGINS] that it was a nice perk, to find that he was the first to gain access to the recreation room, but that sometimes it could be a labour to faze Hercules.

In contrast, for Don Juan deflowering his victim is a *sine qua non*. His layaway plan started with putting a woman down.

Casanova, though, had no attitude beyond the horizontal.

❧ Bad-Girlism

Guys are not the only gender whose love life may get bent by ATTITUDE. Today we observe, wincing, a generation of younger women whose attitude hardly defines the new millennium as MM good.

Bad girls. The image leaps out at us from women's magazines: bold, sneering, patently bitchy broads who have given up on charm, as a feminine asset, in favour of leather pants and persona to match.

Their icon: a chemically blonde singer yclept Madonna — as if the original Mary hadn't already suffered enough. When this trampy messiah — who won notice by performing buckled in a brassy bra worn over not much — finally got married — in an old Scottish castle where the groom could learn how Duncan made a mistake — the event was hailed by her acolytes as the triumph of spit over polish. The massed media gaped in wonder, that virtue could be so resoundingly unrewarded.

The bibles of the bad-girl cult bear titles such as *Bitch: In Praise of Difficult Women* (Elizabeth Wurtzel) and *The Bad Girl's Guide To Getting What You Want* (Cameron Turtle). They extol the benefits (mostly financial) of being hard-nosed from face to feet (in spike heels).

Sartorially, it is difficult to distinguish the film star from a member of the reception committee at a Nevada whore-house.

So, what is the relatively simple-minded Casanovan to make of this new ilk of Amazon, whose unholy mission is to use him for all he's worth, plus depreciation? To be viewed as a utility, like a water main or a street lamp, can be depressing. Especially so as it is obvious that bad-girlism can produce only old girls who have turned their sex's natural milk of human kindness into a rather gamey goat cheese. And crackers.

These bad girls are old enough to know better. And for the Casanovan, unless you are both in the armed service, there is no joy in contributing to the delinquency of a major.

We can only hope, therefore, that as a faith Bad-Girlism will prove less durable than, say, Confucianism, or even Consumerism.

Meantime, a guideline to girls: if it looks too bad to be true, it probably is.

⌁ Bastards

Casanova created a rich heritage of illegitimate children. Both girls and boys. He was not sexist in his generous contribution to the population of Europe. And he was always delighted to meet one of his progeny.

He of course never referred to his children as bastards. In his own mind, every woman he made love to was his wife, albeit temporarily. The marriage might be unsanctified, in fact last only a matter of hours, but in the accelerated time-motion scale of his lifestyle, he saw all his issue as legitimate.

Moreover, the mothers were always grateful for what he had given them: a robust copy of himself. Thus when he encounters Thérèse at a dinner after an absence of years, she introduces him to a youngster of whom Casanova writes: "In whatever he said I was glad to recognize taste, good sense, and intelligence . . . I rose from the table so delighted with my son that I embraced him with the utmost tenderness and was applauded by the company."

Roses are blooming in Bastardy.

Casanova made sure that the blooms he fertilized were well tended: he provided for the mother by subsidizing her marriage to an older man, happy to be dad to a child so healthy though bearing little resemblance. (Usually. Though one of Casanova's bastards actually grew up to look like his mother's husband: the ideal scenario.)

Today's Casanovan has less occasion to meet a bastard, aside from his boss at the office. Sex education being part of the school curriculum, girls are better informed about the conceptual consequences of unprotected intercourse. Also, unwed mothers are apt to feel less charitable towards the fathers. Who rarely get applauded.

Compared to the cordial dinner at Thérèse's home, it is much less fun to be reunited with one's bastard by a court-ordered DNA test. Paternity suits can be arduous. In short, siring bastards has lost much of is innocent appeal.

The condom is a curse on the Casanovan joy of sex. But better safe than sued.

⤳ Bathing

There may have been an occasion when Casanova took a bath by himself, unaccompanied by a woman or a group of women, but his memoirs do not elaborate on the value of mere personal hygiene.

Instead, we get his accounts of bathing as a water sport more spontaneous than, say, synchronized swimming. Casanova pioneered the pleasures of today's hot-tub. Denied the technology of the jacuzzi, he showed that things done by hand can be ultimately more satisfying.

The two operative ways to use ablution as the answer to sexual tension are of course to take:

(a) a cold shower, or

(b) a *bain à deux*

No surprise that Casanova preferred (b). But he recognized the hazards for a couple occupying the same tub at the same time. Such a situation can give intimacy a bad name, especially when a slippery bar of soap is present.

Casanova's solution: to bathe one another in sequence. With the obliging peasant girl Javotte, for instance, he first ministers to her alone in the bath, demonstrating that speed is not of the essence in assuring that all parts of the body are thoroughly laved . . .

". . . My bold hands, running over every part of her body, and remaining more tenderly at some places than others, the poor girl was excited by an ardent fire that was finally extinguished by the natural consequences of that excitement . . ."

Then it was Casanova's turn in the tub, while Javotte — a quick learner when the subject was anatomy — reproduced the rapture in her instructor.

Thus did Casanova raise bathing to the pitch of a Beethoven sonata. With such a prelude, the other movements of the piece built to the memorable climax. Rubber duckie optional.

⬳ Beauty

". . . I beheld a profile at once ravishing and faintly familiar. I attributed that to the idea of perfect beauty that was graven on my soul."

Yes, Casanova was programmed to respond to the physical attractiveness of a woman, rather than the beauty of her soul. The latter might contribute to her spiritual glow but could never entirely compensate for a flat chest.

For the Casanovan, too, beauty tends to lie in the eye of the beholder. The more visually challenged he is, the less he is likely to be vitally disturbed by the profile — head to toes — of a woman seen as beautiful. Buying glasses can be costly beyond what a man pays the optometrist.

"The idea of perfect beauty" is not universal. Among the males of some African nations, and those of the Middle East, the face and figure that the West sees as perfect are viewed as emaciated. That image may be changing, however, as Hollywood's pervasive standards reduce the attraction of sheer poundage in feminine appeal. Rubens is losing ground to *Playboy*.

From illustrations in 18th-century books, we may gather that what transfixed Casanova as perfect feminine beauty was not far off the criteria of men in the new millennium. We share the same conditioned reflex to a palpably healthy woman who offers optimum promise of (a) bearing us bonny children, and (b) providing maximum physical pleasure in the act of conception.

Because Giacomo's own mother was a beauty, embellishing the stages of Europe, he would have been naturally drawn to women of comparable pulchritude. The Casanovan whose momma has depended more heavily on the saw that beauty is only skin deep is more fortunate. His idea of perfect beauty may be negotiable. And therefore he is less likely to be infatuated by the profile of a cynosure thoroughly spoiled by the attention of mind-boggled beaux.

(For the learning experience of being The Invisible Man, the Casanovan need only date a gorgeous professional model. No one will look at him, including her. He has just joined the other trinkets on her charm bracelet — an accessory.)

Yet much as we may acknowledge the fact mentally, such is the power of a woman's beauty that it is hard to dismiss it as "only skin deep." The sub-epidermal values in a woman are to be admired, but the Casanovan responds to what he sees, and with the same mindless lust as that of the highly intelligent, self-analyzing *bon vivant* from Venice.

Cupid, targeting our hormones, makes fools of us all. Aided and abetted by WonderBra.

⌘ Beds

As in Casanova's time, the bed remains the preferred venue for sexual intercourse. This despite the improvisations of people like U.S. president William Jefferson Clinton who are too busy with less important matters — such as running the government — to seek the sack for sex.

The back seat of an automobile, the top of the pool table, or the photocopier — such locales for unleashing the libido may have a certain novelty value, but they always present the hazard of being admitted to Emergency configured like a pretzel.

Certainly Casanova did *his* best work in bed. It was where he accomplished his most amazing feats of endurance. What Charles Lindbergh was to the airplane, Casanova was to the four-poster.

And his 18th-century European bed was primitive compared to our millennial futon and spring mattress. On a water-bed, what tsunamis he would have created!

As it was, Casanova once had to contend with the delicate situation of sharing a hotel bed with the husband of the comely woman he wished to woo, bedded with her sister in an adjoining room. The ultimate challenge: *the bed creaked.* He cannot escape the company of the slumbering hubby and join the manifestly available sisters, without waking Nemesis, who "felt about with his hand, and finding me near him, went to sleep again." Oh, the agony of frustration! After spending much of the night repeating this ordeal: "I had to give it up in despair."

However, "Love is the most cunning of gods." An early-morning street fight wakes everyone up, and while the husband goes to learn the cause of the tumult, Casanova moves quickly: "I am at work while I am speaking. I meet with very little opposition, but leaning rather heavily upon my fair lady, I break through the bottom of the bedstead, and we suddenly find ourselves, the two ladies and myself, all together in a heap on the floor."

When the husband returns from observing the hubbub outside, he finds the ladies laughing amid the debris, and Casanova blissfully asleep in the alternate arms of Morpheus.

DO NOT TRY THIS AT HOME.

Casanova was blessed with luck bordering on the supernatural. The Casanovan should never bunk down with the husband of the woman he is about to have sex with, even though the bed has been approved by Ralph Nader as a safe vehicle.

As for having sex in a sleeping-bag, the horrors are too grisly to be described in a blithe tome such as this.

❧ Bitches

A bitch may be described as a tease with a bad attitude.

In Casanova's time, bitches — both male and female — seem to have been less prevalent than they are today. Women then were readier to accept the hand dealt to them by that supreme bitch, Mother Nature. She who saddled them with menstruation, child-bearing, menopause and physical protuberances that make them run funny.

Casanova got burned by a bitch early on in his career as a fun-loving philanderer. His memorable encounter with one of the witch breed occurred at a grand ball, where a fashionable courtesan of Venice, Cavamacchia, persuaded the young Jacques to go upstairs and exchange clothes with her, as a fillip to the party. When he became aroused by her strip act, the hussy rebuffed him rudely. And later, when they reverted to their own garb, and he was moved to grasp her hand, she slapped his face and threatened to have him murdered if he ever disclosed their prank to their host.

Reflecting glumly on this misadventure, Casanova observes that an honest woman would not so trifle with his hormones. Mean women, he says, are guided by "a spirit of contradiction": i.e., bitchiness.

Thereafter, he stayed clear of cross-dressing with a woman unless she was really serious.

In our time, the Casanovan is not so likely to become involved with a celebrated courtesan with a grudge, unless he works in the advertising industry.

He will, however, encounter the professional bitch more routine-ly. A high percentage of thirty-something women are so bummed out by their experience with men — guys who fail to live up to the feminist agenda — that their main pleasure is to entice at length and reject without warning. Pre-emptive dumping: that is the per-formance of the late-model Bitch.

Casanova's safeguard against a bitch attack was to court mainly very young women (ideal age, fourteen), before they had time to go mean. There was then no law against having sex with a minor — a prohibition that now gravely increases the chance of a man's blundering into the web of a mature female with the mating dispo-sition of the rapacious *Aranea*.

A man today may expect authorities to warn him about an approaching tornado or asteroid, but there is no such thing as a bitch alert. Prepare to take cover.

✑ Boldness

"I met the actress Valville, from Paris, attending a French play and was immediately delighted with her spirited CONVERSATION. The next morning I wrote her a note, beginning 'Madame — I should like to begin an intrigue with you . . .'"

Casanova was nothing if not forthright. He knew that no woman can resist becoming involved in an intrigue, however speculative. The word itself connotes all kinds of goings-on — not exclusively sexual — so that the lady who declines an invitation to engage in an intrigue, with an avid admirer like Giacomo, will spend the rest of her life regretting her discretion.

Valville had more sense, writing back: "Sir — As I have the knack of putting an end to an intrigue when it ceases to amuse me, I have no hesitation in accepting your proposal."

Thrust and parry. The duel of the intrigue is fairly begun. Because Casanova was bold enough to state his purpose. Which was not to discuss the weather.

By his own account, at least, women never took offence at his boldness. He proved that a man's showing his sexual interest in a woman, however frank his approach, is rarely resented. The trick is to avoid the taint of PRESUMPTION.

Cockiness should not be manifest above the belt.

When Casanova "put the hit" on a woman, without a formal introduction, the impact was not compromised by a knowing leer, or the false courage of a few beers.

The apprentice Casanovan is apt to err the other way, leaning over backwards — sometimes literally — not to seem too bold. He may be shy. A pity this, since, with women, diffidence appeals only to their mind. And they are often too busy, in our frantic world, to have time for a man to overcome his bashfulness. He has five minutes, tops.

Indeed, often the boldness of address lies with the woman. We have all seen TV commercials for colognes, the scene on the crowded bus where the perky, pretty brunette ogles the oblivious hunk standing reading his paper, and she deliberately steps on his foot, if not actually leaping to wrap her legs around his waist. But the Casanovan should not depend entirely on public transit.

Nor should he shun boldness in his own approach to a woman, waiting for her to recognize his other virtues. *That* bus just left.

～ Books

Casanova understood the value of books, not only as a reader — let us not forget that he personally debated with Voltaire about the merits of various authors — but as seeker of sexual favours from women. As he reports on his campaign to win the Countess Clementine:

"First I overwhelmed her by . . . purchasing a hundred good books for the knowledge-poor girl, who accepted them with abundant gratitude. No woman in the world can fail to be overcome by being made to feel grateful. It is the best and most safe way to gain ground, though it requires skill to use effectively."

Giving a good book is a doubly wise investment in a woman's gratitude, as it not only flatters her interest in reading but may occupy an evening that she might otherwise spend enjoying the company of the guy who gave her macadamia nuts.

But do not give naughty books. Trying to arouse a woman by giving her the latest erotic novel sold on the Internet by an agency called Smut.com will probably cost the giver brownie points.

Cook books, too, look self-serving. Even worse: books detailing means of self-improvement, physical, mental or spiritual. The woman is perfect, already. The book that the Casanovan gives her merely confirms that *ne plus ultra*.

A book of poetry — a personal favourite of the venereal Venetian — can do no harm, though self-published work is always suspect as having been remaindered, bound for the dumpster.

Giving the lady a book that the Casanovan plans to borrow and read himself — *My Life In The Majors,* by Slugger Jackson, for example — lacks the finesse to which the master refers.

Worst mistake of all, of course, is to give a woman the latest feminist manifesto, with a title like *What Men Want And How To Keep It.* Casanova never had to worry about having his gift book render him neutered.

Today, he would probably do most of his gift-book buying in the Gardening section of the store, and hope that the chapter on pollination titillates the recipient.

～Braveness

"Only the brave deserve the fair." Which also goes for women of colour.

Casanova too has a discouraging word for the wimp: ". . . the charming though feeble sex loves the brave and despises the cowardly. Sometimes they appear to love cowards, but always for their physical beauty. Women amuse themselves with such fellows, but are the first to laugh if they get caned."

Today, in the office environment, women laugh when the coward gets canned.

Despite the promise that the meek will inherit the Earth, the human female, from hat-checker to Harvard professor, still responds to the dominant make when ready to mate. The high-school girl craves the gutsy football quarterback, despite the probability that the class egghead bears superior intelligence genes.

The man in uniform enjoys a clear advantage, unless he's the milkman.

Casanova wore a uniform only briefly, but did wear the badge of courage: his sword. In the 18th century a gentleman did not accessorize his garb with a blade unless he was prepared to use it. Cowards left the weapon in the closet and prayed for no confrontation.

Today, young men try to signal their bravery by wearing aggressive sneakers. Tattoos, too, are supposed to reflect the fearless. But the Casanovan should beware confusing the brave with the merely reckless and stupid. Bungee jumping, for instance, may impress a woman less as an act of courage than as a sign of genetic imbecility. Silly don't sell.

Indeed, with women no longer the "feeble" sex (witness the growing number of female firefighters, cops and pro wrestlers), the Casanovan has less opportunity to look relatively brave. So, he must *not* miss the chance to kill, swiftly and ruthlessly, that spider/mouse/wine steward that has frightened his date.

⚒ Breasts

Not once in his memoirs does Casanova refer to them as "boobs" or "hooters." *Au contraire,* the breasts of his many beloveds inspire him to flights of lyrical allusion . . .

". . . not daring to let my eyes rest upon two budding globes shaped by the Graces . . ."

". . . two swelling spheres more seductive than the apples of the Hesperides . . ."

". . . her snowy breast, which would have shamed the works of Praxiteles . . ."

". . . I have never seen, never touched, anything more beautiful, and the two magnificent orbs of the Venus de Medicis, even if they had been anointed by the spark of life given by Prometheus, would have yielded the palm to those of my divine nun . . ."

". . . I passed my hands over two spheres whose perfect shape and whiteness would have restored Lazarus to life . . ."

"Her neck was exquisitely shaped, and the two globes, tipped with coral, were as hard as marble."

Clearly, Casanova was a globetrotter in more ways than the planetary. Again and again in his memoirs — which could be described as an extended walk down mammary lane — he blames a sublime breast for his being robbed of his reason, and rendered passion's plaything.

Yet he never, right to the end, loses his veneration of the feminine bosom. Was this an infantile compensation for his being ill-nursed by his absent mother? If so, it would explain his telling his pregnant nun: "Let me suck your pretty breasts, as I am your baby." The monastic mom not only grants him this homage but asks to suck his breasts in return — a remarkable scene, by any standard, of bizarre LACTATION.

The reason why Casanova enjoyed this fixation more than with other parts of the female anatomy? He was fashion's fool:

". . . her bosom well-shaped and not large. Fashion and custom made her show half of it as innocently as she showed her white hands."

Women's fashion has only recently caught up with that of 18th-century France. The bosom went into hiding after the French Revolution — one of the reasons why Casanova hated that societal convulsion. Now, however, the Casanovan is exposed to breathtaking vistas every time he clicks on the ruptured rectangle. Lingerie ads beset him in Christmas catalogues. Barely bra-ed bikinis booby-trap the beach. What to do?

Well, he should try to emulate our paragon by respecting, indeed revering, woman's breasts as the most beautiful form ever molded by Mother Nature. Avoid staring, let alone leering. It is easy for the novice's gaze to become lost in an apparently fathomless cleavage, but an appreciative glance must suffice, lest the party buffet be supplemented with a knuckle sandwich.

Think Lazarus.

❧ Breeches

"I have always had a horror of women with breeches, but above all of black breeches." Casanova here records the shock — almost traumatizing — of his glimpsing the underwear of the young lady he was assisting into a carriage.

Autre temps, autres moeurs. Today, few men are turned off by sighting a woman's black knickers. But Casanova made a federal case of it:

"It seemed to me," he writes in his memoirs, "such clothes were a kind of rampart or outwork." He was fazed by the prospect of an impeded assault on the fort. And offended enough to chide the wearer: "This black has filled my soul with funereal images, just as white would have cheered me."

The young lady has enough spunk to tell him that his noting her breeches, whether black, white or polka-dot, was an accident. These things happen, when mixed couples travel in carriages, sports coupes and economy-class flights.

The episode suggests that every Casanovan should examine his own prejudices about women's underwear, lest he be harboring some strange aversion, like Casanova's, that can abort an otherwise promising relationship.

When Monica Lewinsky flashed her black thong breeches at President Bill Clinton in conjunction with the Oval Office of the White House, he was not noticeably put off. It would perhaps have been better for the moral standards of 260 million people if he had been, like Casanova, appalled rather than grateful.

However, it sometimes requires split-second judgment for a man to distinguish the deliberate from the accidental, in Women's book of revelations. These are devious, dangerous darlings, and damned is the Casanovan who would have them any other way.

≈ British

It's a hard question: was Casanova a prodigious lover because he was not British, or is the Briton an inferior lover because he is not Casanova?

The debate still rages. Some historians believe that the English Channel has long served as a watery chastity belt, safeguarding England, Wales and all but the wilder parts of Scotland. If so, the Chunnel may have come too late for sexual adventuring as Casanova understood it.

He did of course meet Britons from time to time, while he was cruising the Continent. These were mostly ambassadors, visiting France to study *la joie de vivre* in case it was infectious.

Fairly late in his career, it was, before Casanova made a foray into

England, specifically London. This was, predictably, a disaster. Desperate for feminine companionship, he attended a performance at London's Drury Lane Theatre, where, on the basis of his rewarding experience with theatre on the Continent, he could expect to meet pretty women. Instead, a riot broke out, patrons incensed because the play was not the one advertised. They tore the place apart. Romance was not in the air, because flying seats were.

Casanova then resorted to what may have been the first gender-specific rental advertisement. He had his house-keeper put the ad in the street-level window of the house he was renting:

SECOND OR THIRD FLOOR TO BE LET, FURNISHED,
TO A YOUNG LADY SPEAKING ENGLISH AND FRENCH,
WHO RECEIVES NO VISITORS, EITHER BY DAY OR NIGHT

The ad drew mostly chortles from the London press, plus many enquiries from very plain women whom Casanova had to beat off on linguistic grounds. He eventually booked in a beautiful Portuguese visitor, who broke his heart when she returned to Lisbon.

What this negative experience says to the Casanovan: subletting accommodation is a mug's way of getting laid. Any landlord will confirm this. It's an ugly segue: "I love you madly, and by the way you're overdue with the rent." Also, the Tenancy Act is medieval in its means of punishing the lease violator.

Much safer is to accost a good looking woman on the street and tell her: "I want you to come and shack up with me so we can have sex on a regular basis. There will be no damage deposit, and you can have a cat if it's been gelded."

As for Britain today, sex is more readily available without a contract, as long as you stay in hotels and don't expect too much from the theatre.

➤ Candles

"At last Nanette, putting on an air of anxiety, tells me that they have no more candle, and that in a few minutes we shall be in the dark . . ."

Guest Casanova does not panic at the prospect of sharing a darkened bedroom with the three beautiful young women with whom he has been making conversation after dinner. He proposes that they should go to bed. In one bed.

"What can we do in the dark?" asks one maiden.

"We can talk."

Casanova was adept at adapting to unlit converse. In such circumstances he supplemented the verbal message with sign language — letting his fingers do the talking. If what they said was ill received, he had the excuse of the imposed darkness.

We tend to forget that Casanova lived in, and profited from, a time when night-hour illumination — aside from the magical moonlight — consisted of candles, oil lamps, flambeaux, fireplaces: flattering light that had the advantage of going out, if properly timed.

Today's Casanovan errs when having an apartment that depends entirely on electrical fixtures, light as relentless as a police station's interrogation room.

Almost as romantically deleterious is his needing to reach a lamp switch from the prone position on a rug, with the attendant dislocation of a shoulder and 911-call to Emergency.

Casanova's womanizing career illustrates the importance of the candle light dinner. With a short candle. Leave the long taper in church. Short and thick, does the trick. And remember to take the battery out of your smoke sensor.

What about the clap-light, the fixture turned off or on by the sound of having your face slapped? Problematic. Even very brief applause can make some women — e.g. actresses — get up to take a bow. The less interruption the better.

Similarly, scented candles, stuck in old, wax-smeared wine bottles, should be avoided, as many women today suffer from allergies, and a sudden, violent sneeze can severely damage a romantic atmosphere.

As for the episode from Nanette & Co., which soon graduated into group sex in bed, Casanova describes the collective groping in the dark as "playing blind-man's bluff." Trust the master to turn that bleak old saw — "All women look alike in the dark" — into a delightful children's game, with giggles galore. Thanks to a provident shortage of candle.

➤ Children

Nearly every man would like to be a father, so long as it doesn't involve raising a child. He senses that, today, being a dad is only one vowel short of being dead.

As a source of heartbreak for the parent, children are second only to the stock market.

No one understood this better than our excessively virile Venetian. Casanova sired dozens of children during his career. Usually he had left town before the mothers even knew they were pregnant . . .

> *He who loves and runs away*
> *misses child support, off his pay.*

Casanova met his children — purely by chance, of course — when they had grown to a manageable age (out of diapers but not yet into debt). Ever discreet, he didn't introduce himself as the papa of the handsome son or daughter he encountered on his return, years later, to the scene of insemination. Even more wondrous, the mothers, happily married to other men who have supported Casanova's kids through the teething and other noisy phases, are always delighted to see Casanova again. Some are ready to repeat the performance, as if the womb were crying "Encore! Encore!"

The one time that this model of fathering broke down was when Casanova fell in love with the ravishing Leonilda, aged seventeen, and had actually arranged a marriage contract when he met the girl's mother, Lucrezia, and was told that he was about to wed his own daughter. A bit of a shock, but no system of paternity is perfect.

The Casanovan who doesn't expect to live his life on the road, as did his exemplar, will need to be cautious about further populating the planet. Even though the state is taking over much of the responsibility for child care, today's father must anticipate the adult child's return to the nest, having flunked maturity.

In short, children *can* be a source of unconditional love, but if the Casanovan just wants someone to play ball with, a dog is compliant and much less likely to hire a lawyer.

⇜ Chocolate

Women prefer chocolate to sex.

Such is the finding of a recent poll conducted by researchers who probably prefer to remain unidentified.

The result would not have surprised Casanova. He fully understood the role of chocolate in giving pleasure to a woman:

"We took a cup of chocolate together, and I then begged her to lie down beside me in bed without undressing." Casanova's fairly standard morning gambit, this, with attractive serving girls, hostesses, daughters of the same, or any beauty in need of a warming beverage.

For Casanova, "chocolate" meant hot chocolate. This libation enjoyed much the same popularity, on the Continent in his time, as Starbucks coffee does in ours. Starbucks doesn't serve at bed-side, however, which is where Casanova found that a cup of steaming chocolate facilitated the relaxed conversation that helps a couple to get to know one another bedder.

Now that we understand the seductive power of chocolate over women, it is all the more remarkable that Casanova did as famously as he did with the sex, deprived as he was of having a pocket charged with M&Ms.

The Casanovan now can avail himself of a vast array of chocs, many of them as decadent as he is. When dining out, he can watch his date's pupils dilate when the waiter sets before her a rich, mocha dessert drizzled with chocolate. He may be disconcerted by her orgasmic cries — "Yes! . . . Yes!! . . . Yes!!!" — but knows that she is not frigid.

Is it immoral to give a woman a box of bonbons on Valentine's Day, knowing full well that you are tempting her with an addictive substance, one that violates every principle of nutrition and dental care, just to facilitate your having sex with her?

Are you putting the Cad in Cadbury's?

Not to fret, Jack. No woman became pregnant by eating a Mars bar. And there are much more deplorable ways of weakening a woman's resistance than with a nice *chocolat au lait*. Go for it!

❧ Clothes

Clothes, Casanova demonstrated, do make the man and, more importantly, help him to make the woman.

Whether he was garbed in the sober vestments of an abbé, or rigged out as the officer in an army with no other recruits, he took care always to present himself as dressed to kill any resistance from fair lady.

He rarely wore anything, however, that could not be quickly doffed, at the wink of an eye, if the eye belonged to an attractive woman.

One of his favourite guises was that of the domino, a loose cloak worn with matching half-mask. This tent could strike in a trice, at carnivals and balls, so that some women were able to recognize him by any part but his face. Smart clothes.

While there were occasions when Casanova was obliged to dress or undress himself, he often enjoyed the Italian gentleman's privilege of having assistance from serving maids. Very young and pretty maids. This service, as often as not, proved to be for the girls a short course in sex education. Casanova was so readily aroused that the discarding of clothes became infectious. He would have found Toronto's Royal York service definitely inferior.

Would Casanova have had such enormous success with women had his stock costume been T-shirt and jeans? Without a doubt. Generously endowed as he was with those aspects of physique that catch a woman's gaze — which rarely focuses on the feet — he would have flourished as well or better.

It is hard, however, to imagine Casanova's submitting to wearing a tuxedo. The decline of the great lover must be linked to this sartorial incarceration. The wedding already being quite abhorrent to the free-wheeling Jacques, the nuptial tux he would have viewed as the costume of the condemned.

His memoirs make no mention of his preference in socks.

As for women's clothes, he had some very strong views. [*See* BREECHES] He hated dress that was too revealing: "I like to see the face and the general outlines of the form and to guess the rest."

"But," argues his fair companion, "the imagination is often deceptive."

"Yes, but it is with the face that I always fall in love, and that never deceives me. Then if I have the good fortune to see anything more, I am in a lenient mood and disposed to pass over small faults."

Casanova would have made a convincing pitchman for Estée Lauder.

Coitus Interruptus

Casanova did not practice coitus interruptus. He didn't need to practice. He came naturally. And often. [*See* STAMINA] Coitus non-interruptus: that was more his forte.

Birth control was not a factor in Casanova's experience with sex. He belonged to the Order of Casual Catholics, and contraception didn't affect his performance in the least. Thus deliberate coitus interruptus occurred only when the lady's husband/father/lawyer showed up unexpectedly.

For Giacomo, the Life Force came without brakes. The many beautiful CHILDREN he left bobbing in his wake across the continent of Europe bore testament to the amplitude of the seed that he scattered with such reckless abandon.

Today the Casanovan, despite the advantages of the automobile, has less latitude for laissez-aller. The paternity suit can punish bad timing, giving him pause at a moment when continuity is of the essence.

Yet what woman is sincerely grateful for an aborted ecstasy? Much as her mind may appreciate the escape from pregnancy, her body will resent her lover's preoccupation with caution. She senses that she has a man who may hesitate to join her in the hot-tub without a life preserver.

And, as often as not, the woman becomes gravid anyway. The alacrity of sperm in jumping to the job ahead must never be underestimated. They can leap tall buildings in a single bound. Many a rueful father will swear that conception occurred although his only ejaculation was "Oh, God!"

The Casanovan will therefore do better — and safer than coitus interruptus — to resort to that other contraceptive device, CONDOMS. With which our incomparable sexual virtuoso was familiar, though not well enough to avoid other consequences that do not need nine months to make a painful appearance.

Doing what comes naturally. Our forefathers, the chimps, had it easier.

≈ Cologne

Lust does have its own randy aroma. But the Casanovan should not, perhaps, depend entirely on a scent easily confused with that of old boots.

If ever a man had a personal scent that women found to be pure catnip, it must have been Casanova. Yet he didn't trust his mighty musk to be effective against all targets. For example, the magnetic nun, Marie-Madeleine, "had, amongst the charms and trinkets fastened to the chain of her watch, a small crystal bottle exactly similar to the one I wore myself." Which "was filled with cotton soaked in attar of roses. I made her smell it."

A great ice-breaker, at a party.

The Casanovan is fortunate that the science of smelling good has progressed beyond the gentleman's needing to carry a little jug of perfume on his watch chain, jockstrap or other ligature. The Calvin Kleins of the new millennium supply their own bottle for their attar of raunch.

These colognes can be so expensive that they constitute an olfactory status symbol. As was Casanova's in impressing Marie-Madeleine with the following aperçu. ". . . the inventor of that essence wears a crown; it is the King of France; his majesty made a pound of it, which cost him thirty thousand crowns."

Chances are the Casanovan will not be able to top that, should his date enquire about the source of his smelling like the Garden of Allah. But he should consider that even the fastest sex pistol of all time knew better than to depend entirely on his own body aroma, armour-piercing though this may have been.

Buying cheap cologne — Midnight in Moose Jaw — may be false economy. The fact that it brings tears to the eyes of the beloved probably means that the stinkum has activated her allergy. She may even stop breathing altogether, clouding your evening with paramedics.

Some guys see all colognes as too sissy to be borne. They believe they can be totally persuasive so long as they have had a bath since the last full moon. It's a gutsy premise, but unfortunately not verified by clinical tests performed in the boudoirs of Venice, many years ago, by the master of manly emanation.

∼ Come-Uppance

". . . I drew her towards me, and begged her to let me give her a kiss. Her RESISTANCE made me angry; and passing an audacious hand under the sheet I discovered that she was made like other women; but just as my hand was on the spot, I received a fisticuff on the nose that made me see a thousand stars, and quite extinguished the fire of my concupiscence."

Casanova retreats forthwith, ". . . as the blow she had given me was but a sample of what I might expect if I attempted reprisals."

There is nothing like a bloody nose to persuade a groper that discretion is the better part of valour. The young lady — whose name, hilariously enough, was Mercy — later apologized to Giacomo, for transforming his beak into a red balloon. But he remained wary of this quarry. Once beaten, twice shy, even for the lover who was the Wayne Gretzky of scorers with women.

The problem: the only difference between groping and caressing is whether the hand is welcome. Sometimes it requires exquisite judgment to know how an appendage will be received. Overconfidence can be terminal. Like the male Ariadne spider, who must pluck the strands of the much larger female's web to lull her into a receptive mood, the Casanovan is courting death. Or at least a jail term for sexual assault.

Today's woman is even better prepared than the maidenly Mercy to deliver a physical come-uppance to him who errs on the side of PRESUMPTION. She may well be a graduate of a martial arts program, adept at kick-boxing that can render a man sterile long after he has been discharged from hospital.

Should, then, the Casanovan ask his date for a clearance form, before he puts his arm around her shoulders? Here prudence must yield to the worse hazard of earning her contempt for any man who lets concern for personal safety control passion. It's a nice question: just how many teeth are you prepared to lose, and still keep smiling?

Casanova's pounded pecker sends a warning: never go too far, too fast. Have a long talk with your hands, before you meet your date. Wear mittens if necessary. Make no move that may be misinterpreted, such as offering to adjust her garter-belt.

If still in doubt, abandon dating in favour of pro wrestling. Less chance of suffering serious damage to your profile.

⇜ Commitment

There are two institutions that require commitment: marriage and the mental hospital. Men have a natural fear of both forms of confinement.

Casanova saw commitment to a woman as a deadly allergen. It made him break out — of the relationship:

"I sent her away without losing my time in promising everlasting constancy — a promise as absurd as it is trifling, and one which the most virtuous man ought never to make, even to the most beautiful woman."

Casanova was committed only to showing a woman a good time, for a short time. Lest she have any illusions about his constancy, he sometimes had sex with two women on the same occasion, in the same bed. His candour did him proud.

For a woman, however, even of today's liberated variety, commitment is apt to be on the agenda of her relationship. Her biological clock ticking faster than a man's, she is motivated to demand commitment because of impending menopause. (The male menopause has no ETA and may not arrive at all.)

Thus the women least concerned about commitment are the young singles (18-25), and mothers (45-90) who feel that they have borne enough children and enough of their father. The career woman in her thirties will have found the job she wants, and has the automobile she wants, and is now looking for the man sturdy enough to drag a baby-buggy up the steps of her co-tenanted house. She will kick your tires, Elmer.

Is then a man ethically required, early on in the relationship, to disabuse the woman of any expectation of his being committed to her? Answer: never. Any attempt to do so invites a slap on the face that tenderizes the entire head. Unless the Casanovan can somehow include non-commitment among the tenets of his religion (Casanovism), he will merely come across as a presumptuous dork, wedded to nothing but an honesty that women find emetic.

No, the kind of commitment perfected by Giacomo was that of friendship. For life. Not with all his loves, but enough to qualify him as a decent human being. He did so by loving with all of his being. Mind as well as body. And with enough intensity of each to make him the constant companion, in her memory, of many a woman, for many a year.

⇒ Condoms

As one might expect, the improved condom was the major contribution of the English to protection from sexual pleasure. Anticipating Britain's Industrial Revolution, the safe found a pioneer in Giacomo. While initiating two young ladies interested in this field of research ". . . I shewed them the little safety-bags invented by the English in the interests of the fair sex. They admired them greatly when I explained their use . . ."

Another argument for private schooling.

Girls today get the little safety-bag demonstration from a female sex-ed teacher wielding a banana. No wonder so many of them are confused when they see the Chiquita presented as neither yellow nor altogether peelable.

On another occasion, Casanova explores his lay nun's writing table, "where I found a box full of certain sheaths preventative against certain to-be-dreaded plumpness." He replaces them with a cheeky poem:

> . . . *Fear not of the outcome to the interior.*
> *Thou canst only become a mother superior.*
> *In the upcoming battle, dread not your defeat.*
> *Merely give a signal, then I shall retreat.*

But she has no faith in COITUS INTERRUPTUS, and quite sensibly (in terse verse) requests the return of her security system. Better a safe than sorry.

Today, the Casanovan may envy such supportive treatment of an object that is (a) embarrassing to buy (all pharmacy checkout staff are female), (b) awkward to apply, (c) an impediment to total pleasure, and (d) difficult to dispose of without violating various laws intended to protect the environment.

Some Casanovans may be bold enough to walk into a sex-aids shop and pick up the latest incarnation of the little safety-bag — textured, clarion-hued, with personal monogram — but they are the exception. A man is more likely to depend on his partner to carry the anti-plumpness packet in her purse.

Women are the more practical gender. That the Casanovan's lady produces a condom out of thin air, like a magician's pigeon, should not be interpreted as the deftness of a woman who has had hours of practice.

Leave the deduction to Sherlock Holmes, lest it be the romance that is arrested.

⇌ Consideration

". . . Soon her sighs and the ardour of her surrender showed me that her passion was more in need of relief than mine. I was sufficiently master of myself to remember that I must have thought for her honour . . ."

Translation: Casanova jammed on the brakes before running her into trouble.

This is the older Casanova, recounting his major affair with Pauline, the Portuguese lady in distress, while both were visiting London. Was his restraint an effect of the English environment, which discouraged the unbridled passion as an aberration from riding to hounds? Possibly.

Another, more likely, factor: Casanova was now into his fifties. It is axiomatic that the older the Casanovan becomes, the easier it is for him to respect a woman's "honour." Certainly when he was a randy young buck back in Venice, Casanova had no compunction about banging virgins, singly or at a group rate.

Today, of course, women have no "honour" to respect. The feminist movement had it surgically removed. Without anaesthetic. Virginity is no longer considered to be a moral asset, for either gender. Sexual freedom begins in high school, where the CONDOMS dispenser in the washroom sets the tone for chastity.

Sounds great, but the reality is that the Casanovan may not have to wait till he goes to Hell, before paying a price for defloration in other than a bed of roses. The proliferation of single, teenaged moms shows up on his taxes, federal and local, as charges for social welfare, even if he isn't sued for child support.

So, consideration is even more pertinent than it was in Casanova's time, when unwed mothers were shunted into nunneries as if their condition were an Act of God.

It took a while for Casanova to mature enough to understand the importance of consideration of the unpleasant consequences for a woman yielding to the passion he engendered. Which is a marker for our young Casanovan, even if his face breaks out from time to time.

Control

"Javotte was not a beauty . . . Her complexion was too sunburnt and her mouth too large, but her teeth were splendid and her underlip projected slightly as if it had been formed to receive kisses . . . I did not propose to make her fall in love with me . . . All I wanted was to train her to perfect obedience, which in default of love has always appeared to me the essential point. True, that in such a case one does not enjoy the ecstatic raptures of love, but one finds a compensation in the complete control obtained over the woman."

Yes, control does eliminate INFATUATION. Without it, a man is apt to find that he has *fallen in love,* an experience comparable to stumbling into a wild-animal trap.

The homelier his woman, the less considerable the threat of competition, which erodes control. And, as Casanova makes clear here, every woman has at least one physical feature that is attractive. It may be hard to concentrate entirely on her teeth. She may wonder why you are staring so fixedly at her mouth, hoping for a grin. But she will blame it on astigmatism.

Javotte was a peasant girl, fairly easy for Casanova to control with his magician act that involved their sharing the family tub, and performing some occult rub-downs. Today, however, girls of all social strata are more wary of being manipulated. The term "control freak" — inescapably pejorative — comes to mind, as a criticism frequently voiced by women describing the husband or lover that they have dumped in favour of a large dog.

"Perfect obedience" from a woman is now but a lovely figment of imagination, along with the foolproof mutual fund and socks that don't shrink on washing.

⤳ Convents

The convent was the source of much of Casanova's early sex education. Marie-Madeleine, the nubile nun who proved to be probably the greatest love of a life that counted many women, testified to the virtues of the Venetian convent.

That institution provided temporary accommodation for what were fortuitously called "lay sisters." The convent enjoyed a surfeit of fat nuns who lost weight suddenly, and dropped the veil soon afterward. As a holy birthplace, it was the manger without attracting as much attention.

The love babies born in the convent were the healthiest infants ever to bounce into a bassinet. True, some of them had to be transferred to orphanages, but others, like those sired by Casanova, were quietly secured a good home by fathers grateful to be let off so lightly.

Instead of condemning abortion, the Vatican today might more constructively reinstate the nunnery as a sane asylum for unwed mothers-to-be. However, the Casanovan should not count on this happening, when tempted to have unprotected sex.

As things are, unless he is flying to Rome on a cultural pilgrimage, he may never see a recognizable nun other than Sister Wendy. Who, though charming, does have that unfortunate overbite.

✎ Conversation

"'I shall always love you, dear Annette. Undress and let us have a little talk'" . . . "Our conversation, taking a passionate turn, lasted two hours."

Every woman finds conversation irresistible. If she can be persuaded to undress before the talk begins, the verbal FOREPLAY complements her state of nature to the predictable satisfaction of both speakers.

Casanova had a special fondness for women who sparkled in conversation. They were inevitably Frenchwomen. Witty. Worldly. Challenging their wooer to hold up his end verbally as well as penilely.

Giacomo always had time for talk: ". . . and we did not find our forty-eight hours together a long time, for two passionate lovers find plenty to talk about since their talk is all of themselves." Through conversation he sought the engagement of mind as well as body, a fusion that necessarily goes beyond the basic hump 'n dump.

One of the problems for the 21st-century Casanovan is that everyone — women as well as men — is so pressed for time that amatory conversation must be accelerated, verging on the gibberish of a rewound tape-recorder.

When we recall that Casanova was conversing in the same era as Samuel Johnson and Voltaire, it is apparent that stimulating conversation of all kinds has since been on the skids. When the woman one is with keeps looking at her watch, or answering her cell phone, because she has an appointment elsewhere, parley poops out.

Another misfortune: some women, especially the intellectuals whose compulsions are confined to the cortex, will insist on talking well into the stage of sexual intercourse when a groan of ecstasy would more than suffice.

In this situation the Casanovan who is not a great talker even when vertical is apt to babble. It tests his ability to be a good listener, occasionally croaking, "You can say *that* again, baby."

It follows that what some men like best about fellatio is that it impedes a woman's talking, at least momentarily.

But the Casanovan should still value the master's example of relishing the conversation that brings lovers together before they are one. Even the cherished one-night stand can be made more memorable if something is said. Besides, that is, "Do you want to use the bathroom first, luv?"

Costs

Every Casanovan should familiarize himself with Woody Allen's immortal bit of dialogue:

"I've never paid for sex."

"You just think you haven't."

The inevitable cost of sex with a woman ranges from that of a tryst with a discount hooker to MARRIAGE — which often means buying new socks.

Certainly Casanova spared no expense in proving to a woman that he was prepared to spend more than the night with her. Granted, the thousands of lira, francs, scudos, roubles that he lavished on women's entertainment were not hard-earned. The gaming table, his potty old patroness Madame d'Urfé, and chancy coups, like his role in setting up the French national lottery, kept him in ready cash that he blew, with a kiss, on the splendid dinners, carriages, gala balls and fine clothes that made so many women much obliged to him. An obligation fulfilled to the complete satisfaction of Casanova and his bankers.

One of the financial deals that Casanova did *not* adopt, despite his rewarding visit to Amsterdam on behalf of the French government, was the Dutch treat. He would not have understood the principle of this confusing of gender roles. The aggressive splitting of the restaurant bill: anathema to the gallant.

Now, it is just possible that today the Casanovan will meet a wealthy, older career woman who is in the market for a boy toy. The dry-land equivalent of a Hawaiian beach boy. Such women are said to exist. Then again, the whole concept may be a myth. Hanging around the ladies' room at the stock exchange could be a grievous waste of life. Be the one to pick up the check, man, and wince later.

Casanova demonstrated that there is no cheap way to prove to a woman that she means more to you than quick relief from sexual tension.

Courtesans

The courtesan was a mistress who had tenure. Casanova's meeting the celebrated and sensationally sensual Cavamacchia, one of the preeminent courtesans of Venice, impaired his budding career as an abbé . . .

"To converse with her, especially to be admitted to her circle, was considered a great boon . . . I found her surrounded by seven or eight well-seasoned admirers, who were burning at her feet the incense of flattery. She was carelessly reclining on a sofa . . . She eyed me from head to foot, as if I had been exposed for sale, and telling me, with the air of a princess, that she was not sorry to make my acquaintance, she invited me to take a seat . . ."

Except when applying to a female bank manager for a loan, today's Casanovan is unlikely to duplicate such an encounter. Indeed he is hard put to find a courtesan equivalent to help him open doors to power as happened to Giacomo, with a minimum of paper-work.

Such is the decline of the sofa, as a power source. We all remember wistfully the portrait of Chateaubriand's "amie", Mme. Récamier, draped fetchingly on a sofa, obtrusively vulnerable, a scene of opportunity not to be found in our time's ergonomically correct furniture. Progress does have its drawbacks.

❦ Cross-dressing

Casanova harboured no prejudice against his dressing as a woman. Whatever it takes: that was his philosophy as a devout libertine.

Usually the occasion was a masquerade dance, a feature of the somewhat decadent social life of the Venetian elite. At one of these incognito balls, in Milan, the affair facilitated his gaining access to the "lovely" Marchioness Q:

". . . The men dressed as women and the girls as footmen. Then it was decided that the costumes of the young ladies were too revealing and might incite all the libertines of the city. Therefore we remained at the apartment I had taken and after removing the unaccustomed BREECHES from the young lady, it was but a matter of a short time before my woman's attire was off and we assumed our rightful relations with each other. She did not remain still a moment, and I have known few women so ardent in their reciprocity."

Casanova was never so fascinated by a woman as by the teenage Bellino, who passed himself off as a tenor castrato though he had "a bosom worthy of Venus herself." When at last this busty boy Bellino surrenders his/her camouflage, the passion of both parties is one that Casanova remembers as one of his finest moments in bed.

Clearly cross-dressing comes in more forms than the Casanovan's trying on his girl friend's black-lace négligée before he wraps it as her Christmas present. And no harm done, as a rule, unless he moves on to stiletto slippers. (Murder on the ankles.)

❦ Cynicism

Despite the high percentage of his multitude of lovers who exploited his perfectly normal male sex drive, to gain benefits besides the erotic, Casanova never became cynical about women.

He entered each new romantic adventure with the blithe innocence of the high-schooler shucking his virginity. If not altogether starry-eyed, neither was he using sexual intercourse as a form of revenge against affirmative action.

When he blandished a woman, the stimulant was sweet wine, not sour grapes.

For the Casanovan today, the motivation may be less innocuous. A gender war fueled by feminism, and the rise of the career woman, have made him prone to the suspicion that the woman who has phoned him for a date is not interested in him only for his body. She may just covet his list of clients. Or his thriving web-site. Or — worst of all — she merely craves a companion since her dog died.

Life for the male libertine was much simpler when women's reasons for compliance were less complicated. Casanova never had to consider that the married woman he was seducing may have read a magazine article written by a female psychotherapist recommending that wives have an affair as a means of sprucing up their marital sex life. No Casanovan wants to discover that a woman sees him as a doctor's prescription. Take one at bedtime. Goodbye divine afflatus.

No such problems for Giacomo. He didn't allow second thoughts to mess with first impulse. In this he could be pure male animal, as simple as billy goat getting his nanny.

Naïve? Possibly. But 'tis better to be madly ingenuous, and enjoy the mating without analysis, than to suffer sudden erectile dysfunction as a result of concern over whether the missionary position represents male domination of women.

Casanova's life was a rosy testament to a man's faith in his pure animal magnetism — insuperable charm — as the catalyst that transformed maid to mistress in a matter of minutes.

The Casanovan should be equally free of cynical assessment. Will he get hurt? Of course. But what's an occasional fatal wound, measured against the bliss of requited love?

ᵔ Dancing

A course prerequisite, for the Casanovan who hopes to graduate summa cum lovin'.

Giacomo studied dancing as a major factor in FOREPLAY. He attended more balls than Yogi Berra. Whenever and wherever in his travels he found himself in danger of sleeping alone, he contrived to get invited to a ball where he could meet, and assess, pretty women. Up close and personal.

The highlight of his visit to Spain, for instance, was his introduction to the fandango:

"It cannot be described. Each couple only dances three steps, but the gestures and attitudes are the most lascivious imaginable. Everything is represented, from the sigh of desire to the final ecstasy; it is the very history of love. I could not conceive a woman refusing her partner anything after the dance . . ."

Obviously more productive than being partnered for pinochle.

Casanova also benefited from the circumstance that the ball was usually held in a great house, with several vacant rooms where a couple could consummate the pleasure engendered on the dance floor. This is where our Y dance, barn dance, "rave" and other venues for dancing lack a vital accommodation. The back of the pick-up truck cheapens the climax of the boogeying.

Yet dancing remains very popular with women, because it affords a woman the chance to judge a man's potential as a lover, without the strip-search. It therefore behooves the Casanovan to learn to dance. If not the fandango, then at least the two-step. The Highland fling won't hack it.

Like Romeo casing Juliet, Casanova enjoyed his time's vogue of the masked ball, which allowed both men and women to flirt outrageously without fear of being identified. Today women wear a mask only to play ice hockey. A whole system of sexual mystery and intrigue has been replaced by the catcher for the girls' softball team. Pity.

Still, the Casanovan should be ready for that rare moment when he may relive something of the glory of Fred and Ginger. In sex, as with other contact sports, much depends on the footwork.

⪼ Dating

"LOVE, INTERNET STYLE, NOW A 'MAINSTREAM' DATING OPTION" (newspaper headline, 2001 A.D.)

In this respect, Jacques Casanova would appear to have been disadvantaged, when trying to get a date. But then he seemed to do very well, romantically, without dating at all. He wasn't dated himself, and he never found it necessary to go through preliminary rituals such as putting an ad in the Personals page of *The Venice Globe and Mail:* "Certified sex pistol seeks company of W, W or B, S or M, for social evening."

Jacques took girls the way Julius took Gaul: I came, I saw, I conked her.

Most of his conquests didn't even know they were on a date till they found themselves in bed with him. They had been lured through the agency of Eros, not Microsoft.

Despite the lack of today's technological aids to dating, such as the Internet, Casanova surfed the whole of Europe, personally, to meet the many, many women who had little warning of becoming his date.

He was as close to being on-line with women everywhere as is possible without a computer.

Casanova, used he-mail.

The disciple who thinks therefore that he can sit on his duff and click on to amatory heaven has failed to recognize the hazards of something called — ominously enough — a Website.

Casanova trusted only his own eyes, ears and nose. A personal approach that called for a lot of travel, as well as having to shave regularly. But he met women fortuitously, out of the blue not the broad sheet.

➤ Debauchery

May be defined as an orgy that leaves a bad taste in your mouth.

Casanova participated in several notable orgies, when he was young and vigorous enough to service multiple partners on the same occasion, in a setting that had its redeeming features. He felt no ill effects. But other times when he yielded to raw sex as a team sport he experienced the regret of one who blames being influenced by keeping bad company:

". . . We went first to one and then the other, and before long they were both in the state of Eve before she used the fig-leaf." After a half-hour of "lascivious combats," Casanova and his friend pay off the girls, "I going to bed cross with myself for having engaged in such brutal pleasures . . . for profligacy depresses as well as degrades the mind."

Now, the Casanovan may argue that brutal pleasures are better than no pleasures at all. Partners who practice group sex in establishments rented for the purpose insist that their relationship is perked up by the promiscuity. But such debauchery would appear to favour the female, who is acting like some tribal chimp sneaking off from the dominant male from time to time, to pick up a few extra genes from the bachelor ape hanging out in a tree made for swinging.

Casanova was the dominant male personified. He was totally uncomfortable with the situation of sharing females with another male, regardless of whether there were enough to go around and the party had some really nice hors-d'oeuvres.

If the Casanovan, too, senses that he will hate himself in the morning, he may be properly cautioned by Giacomo against the debauchery that triggers depression. There are so many other opportunities, today, for a guy to feel disgusted with himself. To go seeking another source of mental degradation — besides watching TV talk shows, that is — would seem to symptomize an addiction to self-loathing worthy of the medieval flagellants.

To Casanova, sex without love was a travesty. True, he could fall in love very easily. In a matter of seconds, actually. And his love was anything but exclusive, if he had several lovers phasing in and out.

By the end of his life he was still deeply in love with dozens of women, most of whom hadn't seen him for years. His was *la vie en rose*, with patches of purple. But a debauchee, he wasn't.

Devotion

Is it necessary to have a long, monogamous relationship with a woman to earn a lifetime of devotion?

The answer — unfair as it may seem to Darby hanging in there with Joan — is No. Casanova proved conclusively that the impact a man makes on a woman can be significant enough to brighten his old age with her LETTERS of endorsement. Huge bundles of fading correspondence with his old flames testify that the great Venetian was not only a formidable physical experience but one graced with the sentiment that endures. To warm him in his grey years.

Writing a love missive to a woman can be the best literary investment a man can make. She will almost certainly preserve his letter/postcard/fax, in some secret place of her heart and even her purse. As Casanova memoirs editor Arthur Machen astutely observes:

"How many more discreet and less changing lovers have had the quality of constancy in change to which this lifelong correspondence bears witness?"

Too few. The provident Casanovans are far outnumbered by

graduates of the Hit-and-Run School. Whose correspondence in old age will be limited to a Christmas card from a realtor.

Their believing that they are God's gift to women will not get the job done, when they donate only their sperm.

So how did Casanova plough so deep as to reap the crop for so long? Obviously he brought more to the encounter than an eager appendage. He *loved* each of his conquests. He was totally focused on that sexual campaign. Nothing else in his life mattered as much as his exchange of intense pleasure with the woman who would remember him, indeed worship him, for as long as she lived.

Casanova *condensed* the devotion of women. In a matter of days or weeks, he planted a radioactive regard with the half-life of a lifetime.

Then what better for the Casanovan to aspire to, than to create for a woman the magical moment, one to recall during her marriage to someone else, less well endowed?

Can he win such devotion with e-mail? Probably not. Electronics favour the ephemeral, whereas handwriting bears the style, the sense, the soul of the sender. The chances that your sweetheart will cherish your computer print-out: poor. Buy a quill, and parchment, and prepare to be remembered fondly by your women, into the twilight years.

❧ Dining

In virtually all of Casanova's more memorable seductions, a sumptuous dinner plays a major role, either as prelude, intermission or — rarely — finale. (Usually sleep takes precedence.)

There is a lesson here for today's guy who assumes that he can initiate a fulfilling affair in a singles bar. A bowl of peanuts simply won't do, as Lucullan feast.

Similarly, despite the regal atmosphere implied by the Burger King, this type of utility trough best suits the married man whose wife has just filed for divorce, or whose doctor has told him to stop worrying about mad-cow disease.

A memorable repast! That is what the Casanovan must provide

for his date. He *could* do this at home, of course, if he is an excellent cook in other than his own mind. But nothing beats a really fine restaurant, as the venue of conspicuous consumption in the cause of coition.

That is, a restaurant that has a maître d'. Or maîtresse d'. Who greets the couple up front, with an admiring glance at whatever one's date is wearing. Try to find a headwaiter who has been trained at industrial school to deliver this flattering though fleeting look that makes your companion feel good about her appearance, though she be ugly as a gravel pit.

Casanova had his dinners catered, or in homes of the wealthy, thus sparing himself the mood-killing intrusion that is presentation of The Bill. Which can trigger contestation by the liberated woman . . .

"I'm paying half."

"No, no! I invited *you!* "

"But I *wanted* you to invite me. I'm fifty-percent responsible."

"No! You can invite me another time!"

"No! I'm getting married next week!"

The ensuing struggle can actually deteriorate into a tug-of-war over the bill, with tableware upset, to say nothing of the maître d'.

Casanova did have the advantage of living in an era when a lady was less assertive about not being obligated to a gentleman. His disciples may be wise to accept "No" for an answer, as it applies to paying dinner bills. No's can be habit-forming. And the only negative that the Casanovan really wants is that of the photo of his charming companion smiling over her just dessert.

◈ Drugs

Casanova had no need for mood-enhancing drugs. He was normally in a mood enhanced to the max. By his own senses of sight, smell, sound and touch. He was on a natural high with women, for about sixty years, a sex addict who went into rehab only at the behest of impotence.

His one experience with snorting a bizarre substance was instigated by a Spanish countess who produced a snuff-box and invited him to a pinch. It gave him a nose-bleed . . .

"There we were, bleeding into the same basin, facing each other in the most ridiculous position." After thirty drops of sanguinary nasal intercourse, this strange woman tells him: "The admixture of our blood will create a sweet sympathy between us, which will only end with the death of one or the other."

Needless to say, Casanova recognized a deleterious side-effect when thus described for him. He hastily moved his nose out of range. Although he later consulted an apothecary, he never did find out what drug he had been induced to inhale. He just made a mental note to avoid Spanish countesses bearing snuff-boxes.

The true Casanovan would not, of course, ever try to slip his date a drug in order to expedite conquest. Just not part of his code of amatory sportsmanship. Here it must be pointed out that alcohol is not a drug, so long as it comes in a shapely bottle with a cork in it. Whose contents are shared. In communion with Nature, or at least some fresh air.

What the Casanovan must beware of is his being drugged by that demonstrably friendly blonde he has met in a bar. Or whom he has become involved with by climbing up balconies. Keep in mind the fate of Romeo dating Juliet. The basic rules of caution:

1. Find out if *her* family has a grudge against *your* family.
2. Avoid setting up a rendezvous in a crypt.
3. Do not become suicidal just because you find your Juliet apparently deceased because of something she drank. She may just have overdosed on daytime TV.

⟐ Dupe

Casanova describes himself as having been "the dupe of women." A victim, and loving it.

The choice for his spiritual heir is between his being the *willing* dupe of women, as was the Master, or a sorehead who expects to get something for nothing.

Casanova saw his being duped as part of the cost of doing monkey business. He could never have afforded to be consistently conned had he:

(a) been married

(b) had other regular employment besides seduction

(c) not been a super-duper himself (befooling men)

"Lucky at cards, unlucky in love." Casanova worked hard at being lucky in both. Most of the time, with success. He understood the dynamics of both girls and the gaming table, well enough to accept the losses so long as they were outweighed by the gains.

As in other enterprises, his profit, as a lover, depended on volume.

The man who puts all his chips on one woman, and is duped, suffers more lasting damage to his ego and/or bank account than he who plays women like the slots (the *one*-armed bandit). The Casanovan keeps moving from game to game, accepting that, at the end of the day, he will be poorer in pocket but richer in memories.

What makes Giacomo an icon for today's often-confused male is that, though often duped by women, he never allowed the experience to disenchant him with the sex. There was no carry-over of bitterness, from one affair to another. No moody shuffling off to a men's therapy group, to stand up and say:

"My name Giacomo, and I'm a woman addict."

"Hi, Giacomo. Have a piece of commiseration cake."

He whose self-esteem is too fragile to sustain his being suckered by a sexy lady has no future as a Casanovan. He should pursue something less risky, like becoming an astronaut.

∼ Education

Casanova was one of the earliest proponents of education for women. Sex education, of course, constituted the major component of the curriculum he pioneered, as a one-man educational facility.

Some of this education was elementary. Basic anatomy. The human reproductive system. (He spared untold numbers of frogs otherwise dissected.)

Casanova was also ahead of his time in relishing the purely intellectual development of the ladies he came to love. His appetite was that of a gourmet, in that he was attracted by the woman of more parts than met the eye.

One of the reasons why Casanova adored PARIS, and had his most fulfilling affairs in that heady city, was that it was already the fulcrum of enlightenment for both sexes. *La Parisienne* displayed a vivacity developed in the previous century's *salons,* where the hostess draped herself on her bed to receive distinguished visitors for an evening of cerebral intercourse.

Hence the story of the Frenchman who was arrested in the Bois de Boulogne for having it off with a dead woman.

"Dead?" the alleged necrophile protested to the cops. "I thought she was English."

Casanova too had high regard for the lively *esprit* of the French-woman. But he was no snob academic. Thus he reports: "I was pleased to educate this young girl and felt that when her mind had been developed she would be perfect." His student, the "enticing fifteen-year-old beauty" Rosalie, is a washerwoman's daughter. For her U. of C. course the only fee she had to pay was sex with the instructor. Private tutoring, on special.

As for his own education, Casanova had little formal schooling after the teenager's aborted study for the priesthood — one of the worst career choices on record. The Casanovan should certainly have more options, even if his university program is based on his taking Women as a major.

He should however remember that attending college is no guarantee of education. In anything. A PhD, for instance, means that a person has worked hard to learn more and more about less and less till she at last knows all there is to know about nothing.

⟿ Employment

Casanova is a model, indeed an inspiration, for today's self-employed entrepreneur. He was his own boss for nearly all his working life, a life that included as little work as possible. One suspects that honest toil would have made him nauseous, possibly spastic.

At no time did he prejudice his career as the world's greatest lover by taking a steady job.

He carried his resumé in his drawers.

As for manual labour, the one time he picked up a tool — an improvised pick — was to break out of his prison cell. A phase only, in a life committed to the pursuit of pleasure.

Casanova's was an unsteady income, drawn from gaming and his occasional gig as a consultant for paranormal phenomena. He planned more pyramid schemes than the pharaohs of Egypt.

Without being an avowed determinist, he understood — intuitively if not rationally — that the gods shoot craps, with our lives on the line. Thus his various risky enterprises made no allowance for a retirement savings plan, other than to die young.

Casanova lived by his wits. Which, as the cyber-gurus tell us, is the formula for success in today's world whose religion is Technolism. The person who has the new *idea* becomes ruler of all that his software surveys. His is the mouse that roars.

The happy part of having your office between your ears — as did Giacomo — is that it liberates the rest of the person to enjoy the fruits of a fecund mind. For our cynosure, those peaches and cherries took the form of pretty women.

It follows that the man who is aroused by office routine, or indeed any kind of rutted industry, lacks potential as a Casanovan. To be a mere dilettante womanizer is far more dicey, as avocation, than loving the ladies full-time, the format of Casanova. It is always the luck of the pure amateur to dally just once with some doll, and incur the paternity suit, or sexually transmitted disease, or arrest for pedophilia, or a ticket for parking in a commercial zone, or all of the above.

The Casanovan, though, is *committed.* The Net sets him free. And the world is his oyster supped from the lips of love.

❧ Encores

"For seven hours, which I thought all too short, we enjoyed one another, not resting except to talk, which seemed to heighten our pleasure."

Sex is one form of expression where a man may repeat himself with good effect. And Casanova could be remarkably repetitive. It is safe to say that, for the woman worshipping his prowess, the second coming was even more awesome than the first.

The Casanovan is rightly intimidated by the master's self-admitted capability to both produce and experience orgasm a dozen or so times in one night, rather than in the calendar year that is realistic for his older disciples.

Every man requires a different time-out to "recharge his battery." If he must — so to speak — leave the power source in the garage overnight, he will disappoint his partner. Women are not battery-operated, orgastically, and are apt to moan "Again! Again!" mere nanoseconds after the man has, in the embarrassing sense, shot his bolt.

Even Casanova was obliged on occasion to create an intermission between sex acts. As he says, his rescue was talk. Mercifully, women enjoy talk almost as much as sex, if not more. But it has to be talk that sustains the erotic mood of the moment. Asking the woman "Hey, how about them Blue Jays?" as entr'acte material — a cold shower, verbally.

Casanova could do the talk as well as the walk. Romantic and arousing. He knew how to put something into a woman's ear besides his tongue (a highly overrated erogenous maneuver).

He did not, of course, reach for a cigarette to extend the recess. Thus avoiding the old gag:

"Do you smoke after intercourse?"

"I never noticed."

Casanova was simply blessed with a sexual organ that was a loyal soldier, ready to return to duty after the shortest of leaves. The Casanovan need feel no shame should he fail to emulate the paragon's feats. His women will be prepared to wait for the encore, if the performance has been exciting and climactic enough to leave her eyes slightly crossed, and her bravos clearly positive: "Yes! Yes! Yes!"

➝ Engagement

Two things may be engaged: the loo, and the lover.

Casanova does not report ever having had a problem with either restriction. He often wore rings, and distributed them freely as gifts to lady friends, but none of them betokened imminent MARRIAGE.

The dictionary, with cold perception, gives two definitions of engagement:

1. a betrothal
2. an encounter between hostile forces

If we include duels under Class 2 engagement, Casanova did become engaged several times. But he never risked his life with a Class 1 engagement. And had he been aware of the complications of being maritally engaged today, the horror of the experience would have made him even more grateful to be living in the 18th century — despite the inferior plumbing.

The torturous ritual of the wedding invitations, alone, is enough to render the fiancé sterile for weeks before the actual sacrifice on the altar.

The Casanovan who senses that he may be falling victim to COMMITMENT should remember that Giacomo too sometimes suspected that he was verging on a permanent relationship. Which, in fact, it often turned out to be — the relationship of old friends who had been lovers.

In other words, he enjoyed *the unspecified engagement.* No vows, no ring, no public announcements or private misgivings. Indeed, Casanova may be said to have pioneered the concept of the shack-up. Cohabitation was not as socially acceptable in his time as it is today. And his experiments with the informal arrangement (mostly at inns) would be considered crude in our day. But the paradigm was there.

Today, a ring may be worn almost anywhere on a person's body — nose, lip, tongue, navel — without permanent harm. Only on the third finger, left hand, does the ring represent the engagement that can change your life.

It is best that when the Casanovan gives a woman a ring, it's on the telephone. The relatively innocuous bedside companion.

◦≈ Eve

Would Casanova have been a feminist, had he lived long enough to witness women's liberation into a wider choice of bondage?

Probably. This man was remarkably enlightened about holding Eve guiltless for the fall of mankind. In one of the most perceptive conversations that he reports verbatim in the memoirs, he has

Hedvig — "the fair theologian" daughter of his pastor host — defend the much-maligned erstwhile rib:

"Eve," she tells the awed company, "had not been forbidden to eat the fruit by God, but only by Adam, and in all likelihood her woman's sense prevented her regarding the prohibition as serious."

Hedvig goes on to cite chapter and verse, quashing her male objectors, to rehabilitate the first lady.

The entire extended debate is suspect, as a vehicle for conveying Casanova's own highly unconventional (for the period) views on matters biblical and the status of women. His goodwill towards gender equality is demonstrated by his subsequently, and simultaneously, having intercourse with Hedvig and her more attractive sister Helen. The man's flair for enjoying both worlds — the fleshly and the intellectual — indicates a generosity of spirit worthy of a Harlequin novel.

True, Casanova mentions no fondness for apples. But neither does he ever resent receiving wit and wisdom from the mouth for which he has other, less cerebral plans.

The Casanovan whose ambition is to find an Eve who will both put out and shut up is not only fantasizing by denying himself food for thought, resulting in a lame brain. He may well find that, like the heady but rather plain Hedvig, the thinking woman is less naturally sensual than the sex kitten who, in Norman Mailer's memorable phrase, "took off her coat as though she was already inserting the diaphragm." But must every dish be apple strudel?

❧ Example

"Though I do not repent my amorous exploits, I am far from wishing that my example should serve for the perversion of the fair sex, who have so many claims on my homage. I desire that what I say may be a warning to fathers and mothers, and secure me a place in their esteem."

To date, there has been no movement among educators to make Casanova's memoirs required reading for parents. A pity, this. A case can be made for tucking a copy of his work (condensed to one pulsing volume) into the Christmas stocking of not only Mom and Dad but of every pubescent girl who has shown heterosexual tendencies.

Or perhaps not. The fair sex has so many other sources of perversion, today, that the book could be redundant, possibly seen as quaint.

So, it is up to the Casanovan to examine his conscience, using a microscope if necessary. Do his "amorous exploits" constitute noxious SEDUCTION, or merely sensible enjoyment of resources made available by the moral tone of our time, namely decadent?

He cannot be held to blame for being born into a period equivalent to that of imperial Rome, with some of Caligula's perversions rubbing off on adult videos.

However, so long as the Casanovan does — as did Jacques — make it obvious that he is a free spirit severely allergic to marriage, blessed or common-law, he cannot be held responsible for a woman's actions. Leave her to Heaven, or to Oprah, whichever comes first.

The Casanovan's strongest ally is the feminist illusion that a woman can have it all: a career, children, and a male consort who will share all duties regardless of any plan he may have had for getting a life. If attractive, her ego will convince her that such sexual favours as she grants him will induce commitment to what she envisions as the consummate conjunction. And, if disappointed, she knows that she can use the ruptured romance as grist for a novel (chick lit).

Fair game, therefore, gentlemen, are the phantasies of any woman over twenty. One of the moral blessing of our era is that it is virtually impossible to pervert a woman. With the abundance of R-rated films and glossy women's magazines, the Casanovan is unlikely to be an example of anything. Except, hopefully, the liberated man.

⬳ Excitement

Peerless player though he was, in the game of love, Casanova never went professional. [*See* GIGOLO] He remained an amateur — in the Latin sense of the word *(amatore)* — all his life. What kept him going back to bed, year after year, was the *excitement* of seduction.

In the social setting of his time, Casanova's reckless pursuit of women was an extreme sport, in that he could have been totalled by any number of outraged fathers, husbands, fiancés, or indeed the women themselves had they not been dazzled by the man's disregard for personal safety.

Because today's women are much less closeted, the Casanovan may never experience the kind of excitement that attended many of the master's affairs of the heart. The thrill of the chase has lost so many of its hurdles that a man's adrenaline is barely tested, unless his deodorant dies.

Gone from love's *carte du jour:* the forbidden fruit.

However, if the Casanovan really wants to feel something of the excitement of flouting the taboo, here are a few of Casanova's tested moves:

1. When guesting at someone's home, make a play for the host's wife/daughter/mother (depending on state of preservation).
2. Case the local cathedral for yummy nuns.
3. Don't hesitate to feel up any attractive passenger (public or private transit) who sits beside you. (Casanova would have really exploited economy-class air travel.)
4. Attend dinner meetings for the specific purpose of playing footsie — ideally with the chair if she's a dish.

Then there's coital parachute jumping. Maybe a tad *too* exciting.

⇜ Exercise

CASANOVA appears to have kept remarkably fit despite a limited range of aerobic exercise. He did a fair amount of fencing, but none of his duels lasted long enough to work up a sweat.

On one occasion — during a visit to London — he was induced to exercise by the Portuguese beauty to whom he had rented room and board and unlisted perks . . .

"She would not believe that love was the cause of my illness . . ." (he had lost weight from sex deprivation) ". . . and urged me to exercise. I took a horse, did not like its trot, urged it into a full gallop and was thrown so violently I thought I had broken my collarbone. When I was carried back to my house, Pauline was so contrite at having been the author of my disaster that she kissed me, and from that moment she was all mine . . ."

As many Casanovans have learned the hard way: exercise performed in order to impress a woman can be harmful to your health.

With his usual incredible luck, however, Casanova was able to get pitched off a horse with the favourable result of his making the object of his desire feel guilty. He had got to first base, and could steal the rest.

This is harder to do at your fitness centre. Falling off a stationary bike, unless there is collateral damage, is not as dramatic as an equestrian launch.

In principle, however, participating in an athletic activity at the behest of the woman you fancy: sound policy. Any resultant injury, whether real or simulated, is likely to make her eager to make it up to you. Kiss it, to make it well. Some very warm therapy has been received in a hospital bed.

It was in bed that Casanova got most of his regular exercise. Since a normal workout could last for hours, in a variety of contortions, he would have strengthened muscles that the Charles Atlas course of body-building never even mentioned. He must have had buns of steel.

Casanova would never have understood the exercise of running, unless he was being chased by some woman's husband.

Conclusion: go ahead and wear those attractive Nike runners, Casanovan, for show if not for go.

ᜰ Exploitation

Is it seemly for a man to take advantage of a woman who has deep pockets, if not other cleavage?

This ethical question bothered Casanova not at all upon his meeting, in Paris, the elderly, still handsome, incredibly wealthy and quite dotty Madame d'Urfé. The lady had a laboratory in her palatial home, wherein an eternal flame burned in a furnace dedicated to transforming base metal to pure gold. Her belief in magic perfectly suited Casanova's talent for hocus-pocus.

"The only course before me," he rationalizes, "seemed to abet her in her lunacy and profit from it."

This he did, for years and years, during which his barmy benefactress sponsored his licentious lifestyle, her letter of credit gaining him admittance to high society and the presence of royalty. *He* turned a woman's credulity into gold.

Today, daffy d'Urfés still abound, thanks to divorce settlements and the increasing number of female bureaucrats and university professors of economics. The enterprising Casanovan thus has ample opportunity to cultivate OLDER WOMEN who happen to be:

- government finance ministers (federal if possible)
- wealthy widows who have turned to a Tibetan religious cult that sees the future reflected in goat dung
- national lottery winners
- lawyers, judges or psychologists.

Not the complete list. Suffice it to say that Casanova would have flourished just as well, in our time, under the auspices of unbalanced ladies with well-balanced investment accounts.

A caveat: the Casanovan should never mix sex with financial planning. Giacomo's relationship with Madame d'Urfé was so asexual, people thought they were married. The lesson is to exploit only the older woman with no interest in having children or any other form of reproduction except bearer bonds.

Casanova enriched his silly sponsor's life with his occult claptrap, without becoming an evil Rasputin. (He would have looked ridiculous wearing a beard. Whiskers tickle without satisfying.)

Exploitation it may be, but what other industry can one say to be as friendly to the environment?

⁓ Eyes

"Men seldom make passes . . ." Dorothy Parker's brittle comment on girls who wear glasses had little relevance for Casanova, who records no romantic interlude in which he first had to remove the lady's spectacles.

He does mention one girl (Annette) who had a minor eye problem: "She was short-sighted, but her large pale blue eyes were wonderfully beautiful." It may be observed that any woman who slid into the sack with Casanova was being short-sighted. But it mattered little to him whether a woman was myopic, since he had no desire to be worshipped from afar.

Anyway, there is no clinical evidence to support the belief that near-sighted females are lustier than those with 20/20 vision. They just depend more on touch.

Is there any difference in the sensuality of women with blue eyes, with green eyes, or brown eyes, or eyes that move independently to watch two guys at the same time? Casanova had an enviable opportunity to make this clinical study, which requires a significant number of participants, but, alas, he seems to have been blind to it.

Thus we must continue to live with the myth (possibly) that dusky-eyed maidens (Latins, Asians, et al) are more readily aroused to passion than aqua-eyed lassies (Britons, Celts, et al). Much of this belief may be attributed to the fact that Englishwomen can experience orgasms without batting an eye.

"I was impressed by her perfect elocution," says Casanova of a celebrated poet he visited, "but she was cross-eyed, as the ancients painted Venus, a mark which I am doubtful the goddess would have savoured if she would ever come down to Earth." He shunned women whose eyes were crossed *before* he had made love to them.

And what colour were Casanova's eyes? Almost certainly blue. Italian or not, this was the only ocular pigmentation to account for his spell-binding effect on women. As with that other blue-eyed Italian, Frank Sinatra, the orbs blew girls away. Rudolf Valentino, the early-days film sheik, had a gaze that burned with a blue flame, as did those two other cardiac-arresting heart-throbs Paul Newman and Robert Redford.

Something about the blue-eyed hunk mesmerizes women, and one has to believe that somehow M. de Seingalt's genes were blessed with a gift from some randy Norseman.

The Casanovan who is not sure what colour his eyes are may mask his sexual insecurity by wearing sun-glasses. Not as effective after dark, or indoors, of course, but always a status symbol.

✑ Feelings

May not be limited to adventurous fingers.

The Casanovan can feel other things about a woman besides —
indeed, instead of — her body. Giacomo himself, despite his libertine spirit, was subject to feelings in addition to pure lust, though
these diminished after age fifteen.

The old man recollects this of his adolescent amours:

". . . a certain dread which today I can no longer trace in my
nature, a sort of terror of the consequences which might have a
blighting influence upon my fortune, prevented me from giving
myself up to complete enjoyment . . . The feelings I fostered in my
youth were by far more upright than those I have, as I lived on,
forced myself to accept."

Casanova concludes: "True love always begets reserve; we fear to
be accused of exaggeration if we should give utterance to feelings
inspired by passion, and the modest lover, in his dread of saying too
much, very often says too little."

With the wisdom of his mature years, Casanova knew that, in
seducing a woman, a man may easily overstate the intensity of his
true feelings towards her. Yet women do not appreciate the consci-
entious measurement of sentiment they inspire. Better to be passion's plaything.

An otherwise promising evening can be ruined for the rational-
ist who hesitates to say "I love you" without first analyzing the statement for permanent values.

When today's woman of the world gives herself to a man physically she is confident that she has enough charm and intelligence
to deepen his feelings into a lasting commitment.

The Casanovan need feel no responsibility for this fantasy. So
long as the feelings that he expresses are honestly carnal, he should
avoid the "terror of consequences" that blighted the youthful dalliance of the grand master.

He who lets his feelings dominate his judgment loves not wisely
but too well. As in all matters of the heart, however, moderation can
be carried to excess. And then who would write the love songs?

❧ Feet

Casanova was a connoisseur of ladies' feet. He had to be. In his time
woman's garb was so voluminous below the waist that often her feet
were the only part of her southern hemisphere by which a man
could judge its topography.

Casanova hated large leg-ends. Accustomed as he was to sweep-
ing a woman off her feet, the less stability she had the better.

He much preferred a dainty foot. Shod in a slender shoe. Which
could be quickly shed for a change of inclination. The Casanovan
is likely to share that prejudice against clodhoppers. Waiting for a
date to unlace her army boots — or, worse, having to do it for her —
slows disrobing at a moment when fingers are apt to be trembling.

It has been said that the reason why men are universally turned
on by stiletto heels (on a woman, that is) on a well-turned ankle, is
that they betoken her willingness to compromise her speed in running away. She is, in a sense, teed up. For the swinger.

However, the Casanovan should not be bigoted against big feet
on a woman. Her feet are one section of her anatomy never suspect
as enhanced by surgery. All else may be mere renovation. Cleavage,
silicon valley. But feet you can trust, even though they do nothing
for your libido.

[Note: toe-sucking, which has had some vogue among members of Britain's royal family, does not appear to have been part of Casanova's amatory repertoire.]

❧ Fidelity

"Regarding Catarina, it seemed to me that an infidelity of that sort . . ." (Casanova had his eye on another ravishing nun, Marie-Madelaine) ". . . if she ever heard of it, would not displease her, for that short excursion on strange ground would only keep me alive and in good condition for her . . ."

The rationale of every married travelling salesman.

Casanova was not of course married to the young novitiate Catarina, but he did refer to her as his "dear little wife." When he met (at the convent) the more mature, witty and challenging Marie-Madelaine, he was moved to put a spin on the concept of fidelity, dizzying in its self-deception.

Or was Casanova making fun of his own rationalizing? Always difficult to tell, in the memoirs of this cunning old goat. A "short excursion on strange ground," although it has the connotation of Darwinian exploration, is an account not likely to impress today's divorce court judge.

For the contemporary man who, on his wife's discovery of the alien black-lace panties in the glove compartment, tells her, "Honey, I was just trying to keep myself alive and in good condition for you" — lotsa luck!

Not being married (by definition), the Casanovan cannot be unfaithful to *his* wife, but may be to someone else's. This doesn't count, as bona-fide infidelity, because he hasn't uttered the dreaded words "till death do us part." Even if a pastor is not staring at him at the time, the Casanovan should avoid speaking that dire phrase.

Other compromising expressions are: "I am yours forever" . . . "There will never be another woman in my life" . . . "I will always be here for you, baby."

The major hazard in these indiscreet avowals is that the Casanovan may, in the heat of the moment, *believe them himself.* Briefly, yes, but long enough for a woman — ever alert for a sign of sincerity — to seize on his words as a symptom of COMMITMENT. Something that he never intended to convey. And before he can ask to rephrase his statement, the woman has leapt into his arms with burning kisses, ardour adulterated by bogus fidelity.

An excellent source of hating yourself in the morning.

What of the girl-friend who is unfaithful to you? Inconceivable as this may seem, it can happen. Minimize the chance by informing your lady, early on in the relationship, that you adhere to an Arab faith that punishes the unfaithful woman with stoning, strangling and stomping on her cell phone.

You may need to wear worry beads, occasionally.

⮞ Forbidden Fruit

". . . the sweetest pleasures are those which are hardest to be won, and that prize, to obtain which one would risk one's life, would often pass unnoticed if it were freely offered without difficulty or hazard."

E.g. Romeo had to climb up that blessed balcony.

If Juliet had been roomed at ground level, or living in a walk-down flat, the pleasure won by Romeo would never have tasted so sweet. To add to the sucrose content, he dared to attend the masked ball at the Capulet house. He risked his life again and again. Juliet could hardly fail to be impressed. And Romeo did win a few hugs, before he tripped over a tangled plotline.

Casanova, too, attended his share of masked balls where his life was on the line. Unlike Scott's Lochinvar, he never had to ride off with his prize on horseback, pursued by a posse of angry relatives, but he did have some dicey passages in gondolas, stage coaches and shaky ships that added zest to his eventual liaison with a lady.

Today, the Casanovan is offered fewer opportunities to enjoy the special thrill of romantic conquest despite impossible odds. Not only is the game played on a level playing field but nothing is out of bounds.

Hence today's short list of "pleasures hardest to be won":
1. Seducing a beautiful, middle-aged virgin who is an executive in the government's department of women's affairs.
2. Sex in the bucket seats of a German-made SUV.
3. Fellatio with a lady armed with a really serious over-bite.

Foreplay

Is not a matter of yelling "Fore!" before playing around.

Casanova well understood the importance of foreplay, as a prerequisite to mutually pleasurable intercourse. Although some women are "hot to trot," and actually startle younger men in their eagerness to set a new record for shortest time between eye contact and orgasm, these are in the minority. It's a prostitutional performance and, in a non-hooker, indicates a psychotic condition inimical to true romance.

For loving that is more than mere relief from sexual tension — Casanova's preference throughout his career as a libertine — the male partner must be prepared to invest time and a measure of restraint that makes his knees jitter uncontrollably, unless firmly crossed. As with the delectable Marie-Madelaine:

"As a lover respectful, tender, but bold, enterprising, certain of victory, I blended delicately the gentleness of my proceedings with the ardent fire which was now consuming me, and stealing the most voluptuous kisses from the most beautiful mouth, I felt as if my soul would burst from my body. *We spent two hours* [italics added] in the preliminary contest, at the end of which we congratulated one another, on her part for having contrived to resist, on mine for having controlled my impatience."

Casanova put in hours of foreplay in various forms — including expensive dinners, luxury accommodation, stroking her ego — before he finally consummated his love for Marie-Madelaine. With whom he fashioned the warmest and most durable relationship of his exemplary life.

For the Casanovan who has no natural aptitude for foreplay, there are a plenitude of manuals that detail the effective steps to arousal in a woman. He should not be discouraged to learn that the preliminaries are so much more demanding of patience than, say, priming a stove, or fly fishing.

An even more reliable source of data about foreplay mechanics is today's Harlequin novel. Phrased to create a vicarious turn-on for the female reader, the graphic descriptions in these randy works are said to leave nothing to the imagination. As such they should serve as a useful corrective for the novice Casanovan whose notion of foreplay consists of enthusiastic groping, within the limits of the handcuffs.

Making love to a woman is an art, not a sport. Woe to him who fails first to remove his Nikes.

➣ Fortune

"I was then forty-nine and expected no more of fortune's gifts, as that coy and capricious deity loves and favours only the young and abhors those of ripe years."

Casanova did not actually retire from romancing the fair sex at forty-nine, but he did realize that he could no longer afford it, on the lavish scale of his first half-century.

He who lives on his wits eventually loses support.

On the other hand, even for the man who has not leaned on fortune, but has spent his younger years with nose to grindstone, and the other sensitive appendage restricted to spouse, life after fifty is a downhill without the fun of schussing.

Youthful dalliance is bought at the expense of the senior's financial comfort. Yet the man who adulterates his dedication to loving women by adoring his mutual funds, or by wooing promotion at the office, is not a true Casanovan. He is an amatory dilettante.

Women have no use for such a man, except to marry.

Luckily for the Casanovan, Dame Fortune smiles more broadly on women today than in Giacomo's time. She is less sexist. This is evidenced by the growing proportion of the female population — in the West at least — that is financially independent, without having to wait till Daddy's will is probated.

Although there are fewer royal courts for him to exploit than in the 18th century, the reincarnated Casanova is blessed with an abundance of romantic venues in which to meet and seduce fortunate young women: ski villages . . . scuba diving clubs . . . dude ranches . . . fitness centres . . . investment clinics.

The financial emancipation of women has been a godsend to the Casanovan astute enough to take advantage of it. The downside: young women have even less use for an aging Lothario than in the days when he was needed to rescue them from ill fortune. He can always find a solace of sorts on the links, of course, but it may have to be as a caddy.

Fortune is still the bitch goddess.

~ Freedom

"I have loved women even to madness, but I have always loved liberty better."

The aging Casanova here summarizes his priority. His comment is inspired by remembering a brush with wedlock that happened long after his being able to blame it on youthful indiscretion:

"Twelve years ago, if it had not been for my guardian angel, I would have foolishly married, at Vienna, a young, thoughtless girl, with whom I had fallen in love."

Giacomo's guardian angel was worked overtime, and with a dubious mandate, in preserving this womanizer's freedom. Obviously age does not reduce the hazard. Young men and women today can "love to madness" without a thought of matrimony. But after thirty, both genders are subject to a desire for continuity in a relationship, if only because the restaurant bills are menacing their RSP.

Even the most rational man may feel the sudden urge to "settle down." Sometimes it happens when he wakes up in the morning and finds that he is still alone in bed. His evening prayer has not been answered, because there was no mention of MARRIAGE. He faces another day in solitary. Possibly *alone in a crowd* — the worst kind of loneliness — surrounded by other people from whom he can expect nothing but an airborne infection. Like, road rage.

Freedom palls most quickly for the man who lives in an apartment building that doesn't allow pets, regardless of leg count. No horse. No dog or cat or even a love bird that has been neutered. Result: he starts thinking human company, big-time.

This is why we find more same-sex couples — at least one of them a guy — cohabiting in the big city than in the country, where a guy can find at least some degree of companionship with a raccoon.

Even our desperately heterosexual Casanova wannabe may be swayed by Beatle Paul McCartney's famous dictum: "Freedom is having nothing left to lose." Living up to that credo, McCartney married. Only to have his wife predecease him. Fate *imposed* freedom on Paul, a fate that Jacques nimbly evaded.

True, we may consider Casanova to have been a prisoner of his own libido, but as correctional institutions go, it was of the best.

Free as the breeze — at least till the wind died down — Casanova was a tireless traveler of the western world. The moving target, hard to hit with a wedding vow. A natural law.

Call it The Statute of Liberty.

⇝ Friendship

"A Platonist who pretends that one is able to live with a young woman of whom one is fond, without becoming more than her friend, is a visionary who knows not what he says."

Two can live as cheaply as one, but not as chastely. Or put otherwise: absence makes the heart grow fonder, and also cools off the gonads.

Despite the warning from the Venetian expert on gender relations, the Casanovan may, in the innocence of youth, or the senility of age, persuade himself that the platonic relationship is feasible with a pretty woman who shares the accommodation.

He has forgotten (if he ever knew) the stark stat: virtue is 90-percent lack of opportunity.

Evolution has granted man five senses: sight, smell, hearing, touch and taste, any one of which, operating in continuing proximity to an attractive female, is powerful enough to overcome the most carefully considered resolution of a potential saint.

Most men recognize the frailty. When they shack up with a woman, they concede the likelihood that they will become something more flammable than friends. She will become that clumsy designation: his "significant other." Such a status did not exist in Casanova's time. Between "wife" and "mistress" there was no category for the female pal who expected him to share the making of breakfast.

For Casanova, the problem was with his housekeeper: "too young, too pretty, and above all too pleasant, she had too keen a wit, for me not to be captivated by all these qualities conjoined; I was bound to become her lover."

Moral: never become too friendly with your housekeeper/ landlady/ letter carrier/ cleaning woman, or *any* comely person whom you see on a regular basis.

Women are not looking for a male friend who will become nothing more. When they want a friend, they enlist one (or more) of their own gender. The reproductive imperative is too strong for *their* best intentions, too, so that the delusion is mutual.

Casanova avoided the hazard of the friendly housekeeper by not having a house to keep. (Except once, in Paris, when he got carried away by wealth.) He kept moving, mostly from inn to inn, or to someone *else's* house (preferably a palace), where he could concentrate on the host's wife or daughter without becoming a friend — bosom, trusty or fast.

The Casanovan's best friend is his tote-bag.

~ Frustration

"NO, no! Put your arms down. If we can kill each other with kisses, let us kiss on; but let us use no other arms." [Clementine]

Occasionally Casanova encountered a virgin whose will was all won't. One stronger than his will to win. He suffered the agony — worse than psoriasis — of *frustration*.

No-hands kissing can be even harder on the body than no-hands riding a bike. Being denied use of the arms, including the short arm, pretty well eliminates hugs. Yet the feet, alone, are not going to get the job done.

Casanova reacted badly to maidens who balked:

"The situation in which I found myself is impossible to describe. I deplored the prejudice which had constrained me, and I wept with rage. I cooled myself by making a toilette which was extremely necessary, and returned to my room."

Round 2: Clementine comes out of her corner feistier than ever. He hasn't laid a glove on her, and is still sucking air. She counter-punches:

"I am full of the poetic frenzy and prepare to tell the story of the victory we have gained in verse."

Instead of having sex she's aroused by the idea of writing a poem about how they both won out over lust. Victories don't come any more pyrrhic than that won by the frantic Jacques . . . "I suffered a dull pain in the part which prejudice had made me hold prisoner while love and nature bade me give it perfect freedom."

Even in our era of sexual enlightenment, the Casanovan may encounter the prejudice that gave our great freedom fighter such an awesome ache in his drawers. Once a virgin — or, worse, one who isn't — sets the bar that high (marriage or zilch), he can expend enormous energy butting his head, and other prime appendage, against a stone wall.

Casanova was so besotted that he took Clementine and her entire family to Milan for a holiday, all expenses paid. He did finally overcome her "prejudice," and they became exemplary lovers. But the cost in time and treasure suggests that what he bought was no bargain.

So, the Casanovan who meets frustration should be somewhat comforted by the thought that even the world's most eminent lover had episodes of penile constriction that brought tears to his eyes. [*See* NO!]

Don't put all the blame on bad breath.

⟨⟨ Games

Strip poker is of course the game of choice, for the man who aims to abridge the interval between introduction to a lady and wild sex. But the card game always poses the chance of his losing. He risks going home in his drawers (or less), with nothing to show for his evening except his opponent's promise to let him have first bid at her rummage sale of his apparel.

Casanova never mixed card games with the game of seduction. He preferred the outdoor pursuit of coy female by ardent male, without falling over house furniture. When he deliberately lost the race, he had to pay a penalty . . .

". . . to find her ring, which she has hidden about her person. We sat on the grass, I visited her pockets, the folds of her stays, of her petticoat; then I looked into her shoes, and even at her garters . . . I was of course bound to discover it. My reader has most likely guessed that I had some suspicion of the charming hiding-place in which the young and laughing beauty had concealed the ring, but before coming to it I wanted to enjoy myself. The ring was at last found between the two most beautiful keepers that nature had ever rounded."

Such is the game as a type of FOREPLAY. Hide and sex. It is probably most effective with younger women who get an adrenaline rush from being chased, and works for men who still remember the thrill of finding the Easter egg in the park.

The Casanovan may find aquatic games to be an equally beguiling prelude to intimacy. Some women, frolicking in pool or lagoon, seem to see phallic promise in the approaching snorkel of a skinny-dipping male.

For the older but still game guy, the hot-tub is said to provide a venue for less physically demanding games (bare footsie), though the chance of drowning is still there.

The bottom line for the Casanovan: do not rely too heavily on chess, as a game that leads to amatory adventure. That contest is too cerebral, and calls for too much checking, before you get to mate.

⌘ Garlic

". . . Then I ordered all the family to kiss me, and finding that Javotte had eaten garlic, I prohibited its use by the entire household."

Casanova's ban on the bumptious bulb suggests that he abominated garlic breath, as a form of bio-terrorism. At the time of his prohibition of use of the clove from Hell, he was the guest of the family of the juicy Javotte, all of whom he was trying to impress with his powers as a magician.

He apparently did not use garlic-modified expiration as a way to sweep a girl of her feet.

Today, garlic breath is almost the norm, for couples who dine out a lot. Since they share the same effluvium, it is only the innocent bystander who reels. Some restaurants require the dinner host to sign a waiver, to disclaim responsibility if his guest exhales.

Some guys use garlic in their pre-date meal, being under the impression that garlic boosts the sex drive into cruise gear. They probably confuse garlic with ginseng, the man-shaped root that has allegedly helped to make China the most populous nation on earth without making people's eyes water.

Some women also take garlic for medicinal reasons. E.g., they are trying to get rid of a relationship. No need to cheat on their husband to get a quick divorce. Just cook up a livid lasagna, then dare him to come to bed.

Five ways that the Casanovan can tell that his garlic-seasoned home cooking has proved offensive to other humans:

1. When he enters an elevator, the doors refuse to close.
2. His canary dies.
3. His house is surrounded by an emergency response team.
4. His breath mint tries to crawl out of his mouth.
5. His girl friend has trained herself to put on a gas mask in three seconds flat.

If it is the lady whose garlic breath withers his lust, the Casanovan should contrive to meet her on a wind-swept cliff. With a breath-taking view.

❧ Generosity

"There can be no doubt that kindly and generous feelings are more often to be found in the hearts of women than of men."

This gracious generalization is offered by our elderly memoirist, who has the credentials to judge the relativity of male and female generosity. Yet elsewhere he observes wryly that, life-long, he has ever been "the dupe" of women. If women are the sweeter gender, why does our guy sport all those bruises on his memories?

The answer has to be that women show kindly and generous feelings towards all living creatures except spiders and men who also move too fast.

Is it not significant that nearly all our animal shelters are run by women? If you are a wounded barn owl, the person who nurses you back to health is not likely to be a heterosexual male.

Casanova himself was nursed back from what he thought was to be his death-bed, by a veiled mystery woman whom he discovered later to be a former lover. The inference: when healthy in bed, he treated women with the total attention to detail that encouraged them to be generous.

The message: It is not smart to dump a girl who may later turn up as your nurse after you have had surgery. To be catheterized by a former lover with cause for resentment is not a fate to be recommended, unless your post-op breathing will benefit from prolonged screaming.

Also worth remembering: woman is the more generous sex in spending time and money to make herself attractive for a man. From her expensively-coiffed head to her pricey high heels, she donates to his pleasure. And it isn't even tax deductible.

When her natural generosity is betrayed, a woman scorned may be transformed into the Hell's own fury of a bitter feminist. But such feminism, like death, is an acquired trait. To live and love in fear of it is to lose much of what a woman has to give.

Bottom line: inside every militant feminist is a kindly, generous woman screaming to get out. Listen closely, with your head on her heart, and you shall hear her.

☞ Genitalia

The word suggests the name of some exotic, semi-tropical isle. Genitalia. A lush paradise of coconut palms, where gentle, dark-skinned maidens sport in pristine waters. Ah, Genitalia!

Despite the romantic connotation, Casanova doesn't use the word much in his memoirs. "Do not call things by name," he was told by an old and apparently wise lady, when he was only twenty and receptive to advice to the lovelorn.

Result: Casanova is the master of the genital euphemism. Always elegant. He never refers to "her whatsit." Or "thingummy." His love's vagina becomes variously "the temple of Venus" . . . "the sanctuary" . . . "the gem" . . . and the hallowed "other that."

This shrine is garlanded with "ebony fleece." It is also a basilica whose portal is parted so the invader may pillage "the chamber of love."

Giacomo is somewhat less reverent when alluding to his own genitalia. His penile pilgrim becomes "the steed" . . . "lightning" . . .

"the little chap" . . . "the masked bandit" (when condomed).

Oddly he never gave that vital organ a Christian name, as do many lesser men who see it as their closest companion. Perhaps this was because a cognomen — Willie . . . Jocko . . . Rover, etc. — would somehow trivialize the creator of so much shared rapture. "Sir Always Willing" has a loftier sound. At times, of course, when knighthood is in flower.

Whatever name the Casanovan chooses, the christening ceremony should be private.

~ Gifts

For most men, buying clothes as a gift to the woman in their life is the supreme sacrifice. Comparatively, getting killed in a duel over her is easy. A man would sooner cross a battlefield under fire than walk into the lingerie department of a store.

Women know, or at least sense, that the ordeal has been suffered by their lover to please them. And the reward is commensurate with the severity of his anxiety attack.

This principle was well understood — almost intuitively — by Jacques Casanova. When he meets the incomparable Henriette, who is travelling disguised as a Hungarian army officer, he spares no expense to outfit her with all the garments needed to confirm her gender. "Dresses, caps, mantles," he recalls ordering from the hosier, "in fact everything, for the lady is naked."

Gutsy stuff. Bold delivery, and no fumbling for a shopping list. He adds: "She is my wife."

"Ah," says the merchant woman, "may God bless you! Any children?"

"Not yet, my good lady, but they will come, because we do everything that is necessary to have them."

Now, that is the way to deal with the female clerk at Sears. Casanova could lie like a sidewalk, if it got him better service. "I took the best of everything."

Rule for the Casanovan: the sensibly priced gift is worse than no

gift at all. Whereas he who gets carried away at the cashier, yet shall
he be transported in bed.

≈ Gigolo

When he was about sixty, and almost ready to retire from active service against maidenhood, Casanova encountered an Englishwoman
who shocked him — no mean accomplishment — by offering him a
job as her paid lover, with a four-year contract signed and sealed
with a kiss.

Casanova balked. Although he was rapidly running out of rich
patrons, and could well use the money, apparently his manly pride
couldn't swallow the role of gigolo. Or, it may have been the fine
print of the contract, which stipulated a trial period of time trials
before the English lady finalized the deal.

Or, again, she may have had a physical aspect as off-putting as
her morals. (The British female can have equine features that
make sex highly dependent on the lover's meeting her in a stable.)

Whatever, Casanova's outrage does him credit. He may have
accepted little remembrances from some of the hundreds of
women he delectated on the divan, but he drew the line at the bil-
let due that had to be notarized.

Today, it is the older career woman that the Casanovan must be
on his guard against, whether English or horseless, if she seeks to
engage him as a boy toy. It is said that the beach boys of Hawaii sup-
plement their income by gratifying wealthy vacationing American
women who aim to explore something younger than Mauna Loa.
For most guys, however, such employment is not something they
would care to include in their resumé. Foolish, macho pride it may
be, but Casanova set the example for the rule:

Wherever else you put it, never put it in writing.

≈ God

"Trust to me, and be quite certain that God has sent me on your way
to assist you."

Thus Casanova, by way of reassuring the beautiful countess in distress, whom he has picked up at a Venice gondola stop. Giacomo is not shy about getting a referral from the Almighty, to facilitate a romantic operation.

Does this mean that his relationship with God was somewhat more opportunistic than that of, say, the pope? That depends on which pope we are discussing. But a reading of Casanova's memoirs does leave one with the impression that, for this adventurer, the supreme being was Lady Luck. Had he not been more usefully occupied most of the time, he might have developed a formal philosophy of determinism more consistent than his forays into the laws of chance to develop the national lottery of France.

Casanova's early unfortunate experience as a teenage abbé — getting tipsy and garbling his homily before a full house of worshippers — may have been a factor in his viewing God's commandments as more of a menu. From which he chose to observe all the injunctions except those against killing, adultery and coveting just about anything that promised to be fun.

His God was Pleasure. And he sacrificed himself, body and soul, in his devotion to that deity. True, he did make a major contribution to Italy's nunneries — mostly in the form of girls he had made pregnant — but none of his extended, lifelong pilgrimage was made to any shrine but a damned good time.

No, Jacques was not an atheist. He was too busy living the good life to formulate a serious disbelief in God. He was willing to leave God undisturbed, so long as God didn't interfere with his plans for the evening.

It follows that the potential Casanovan should examine his own fear (if any) of God, before telling any of his new female acquaintances to be assured that the Creator has sent him to assist her. To be suddenly assaulted by thunder and lightning during an outdoor seduction might faze him more that it did the consummate lover. Who neither blamed Divine Providence nor thanked Her for ideal conditions, being an 18th-century classicist whose first loyalty was to Venus.

Casanova spent many hours on his knees, before what he called "the temple." But his place of worship may not be compatible with that of the Christian who communes only on Sunday.

To each his own epiphany.

∽ Gondolas

The gondola may be defined as a canoe on steroids. But it is more. Scholars disagree on how much influence the gondolas of Venice had on Casanova's development as the greatest sexual athlete of all time. Most would concede, however, that the vehicle has been more conducive to romance than most public transit, such as bus or underground. Unlike today's taxicab, the driver usually was *behind* the passengers of the gondola, who were free of concern about a rear-view mirror.

At one point in his carnal career, when Casanova was carrying on simultaneous affairs with two charming novitiates of the nunnery on the lagoon island of Murano, he commuted by gondola and employed this silent love boat to convey them to assignations in the city. Because the water there can get rough — Casanova nearly drowned in a storm, a human sacrifice to Eros — the gondola signified the intensity of his ardour for these women. Who of course rewarded him more generously than if he was accessing them in a Ford pick-up.

Also, his hands were free. As he reports of an evening at the opera with an officer and his attractive female companion, when he gives them a lift home in his gondola:

"Thanks to the night's darkness, I gained from this pretty woman as many of the favours as can be granted in the company of a third person . . ."

All the perks of a limo. Supplemented by watery street lighting. Just a couple of the benefits denied to the 21st-century man living in the canal-challenged cities of America.

But shame on the Casanovan, if he uses the paucity of gondolas as excuse for failing to make the most of transportation. Without, that is, having to park first.

Since driving a car one-handed is an invitation to brief ecstasy only, and not recommended by the CAA, he may need to hire a punt.

So weep not for the loss of the gondola, you not of Venice. The vehicle does have its drawbacks (e.g., no airbags). And gondoliers have gone union.

⤳ Hair

". . . Bettina groomed me each morning. She would comb my hair, often before I was out of bed, saying she had no time to wait until I was dressed."

It is fair to say that maid service has gone downhill, since Casanova did his guest bit. Bettina, the "pretty, lively" thirteen-year-old sister of the teenage Giacomo's mentor, Dr. Gozzi, was soon taking care of other hirsute areas of the lad's anatomy.

Such hairdressing was a grooming perk for which Casanova benefited often in his career. His portraits show him to have had luxuriant locks, styled in a combination pompadour (pioneered by the mistress of Louis XV and good friend of our hero), and what we now call a pony-tail, though such an equine connotation would have shocked the elegant Venetian.

The Casanovan, whatever his thatching, is likely to have his hair tended to by a stylist who doesn't make bed calls. If hard-pressed financially, he may be shorn by a common barber, male, and even less apt to take heroic measures to earn his tip.

Whichever, his attractiveness to women is inordinately dependent on his having head hair of *some* kind. A bald Casanova is inconceivable. No woman yearns to run her fingers through your scalp.

What about a wig? Certainly this resource was widely used by gentlemen of the 18th century. Today, however, wearing a rug must be seen as a last resort, for the Casanovan. Vigorous sex can be sadly compromised if your piece flies off without warning.

Similarly, the Casanovan who emulates his idol by pumping a pomade into his crowning glory must take care not to overdo. The gunk's purpose is to titillate the lady, not overcome her with fumes. And gentlewomen *don't* prefer blondes.

∼ Happiness

Can a heterosexual man find happiness, without the company of a woman?

The obvious answer: Yes, but it puts a lot of weight on his golf bag.

Nor should happiness be confused with the brief euphoria of intercourse. Casanova (an authority on the subject) makes this clear:

". . . by allowing after each pleasure the calm which ought to follow the enjoyment of it, we have time to realize happiness in its reality . . . those necessary periods of repose are a source of true enjoyment, because, thanks to them, we enjoy the delight of recollection which increases twofold the reality of happiness."

Thus the man who treats sex with a woman as a hit-and-run accident is not apt to derive happiness from the collision. If very young and virginal, he may feel a sense of relief, as when the cricketer has "broken his duck." But happiness? Not likely. It takes a mature lover, like Casanova, to savour the experience, rather than just feel dirty, as will happen after that hectic episode on the pool table at a friend's house-warming party.

At the other extreme, a man may spend a lifetime vainly seeking happiness with the same woman. This makes him a *spouse. Spouse* is not a word that evokes hope of happiness. *Spouse* rhymes with *mouse, house, grouse, souse, louse* — words that strike the ear with the flat of the hand.

The spouse who manages to overcome this handicap does, of course, attain the greatest happiness of all: that of being partner in an old and affectionate married couple. But that may be more than the Casanovan dare aspire to. Unless, that is, he takes early retirement from philandering. With the institution of marriage threatened by the social revolution that renders it an obsolescent device for the procreation and rearing of children, Casanova's model of happiness becomes the paradigm.

This shuns promiscuity — the quick fix — in favour of a relationship that is happily nurtured till circumstances require a reluctant farewell.

Such happiness provided the aged Venetian with the memories to keep him warm. No substitute for having a younger, adoring wife, perhaps, but fantasies are for Disneyland.

⟿ Harlots

Demonstrably oversexed as he was, Casanova sometimes had to resort to "ladies of the pavement." They were not his preference. Usually they served to release sexual tensions built up in pursuit of more challenging quarry that somehow escaped his grasp.

In his snit fit he might take on the entire staff of a brothel, simultaneously, creating enough laughter to cool out his concupiscence.

It has been sagely said that — the rapist excepted — every man pays a price for having sex with a woman. The cost may be as little as a burger for two at Wendy's, or as much as MARRIAGE, parenthood and the 25-year mortgage.

In Casanova's Europe, the spectrum of bought carnal benefits ranged down from the mistress (of king, cardinal, or other successful entrepreneur), to courtesan (of a select club), and the lowly harlot (the common man's social worker).

It was also pretty well understood that any woman appearing on the stage — with the possible exception of the opera's fat lady — was a dancer with more moves than the critics observed. Hence our hero's fondness for the theatre. Between the ballerinas on stage, and the bored, wealthy and attractive wives in the box seats, Casanova nearly always has an excellent selection of romantic objectives. Without plundering his purse.

It was only when cruelly thwarted by fate that he resorted to the common bawdy house. And, to his credit, he hated himself in the morning.

The Casanovan may feel that some self-hatred must be borne to avoid the facial twitch's spreading to the entire body. However, our social conscience has been refined, since Casanova's time, to create contempt for the john. He would never cruise the stroll to pick up a hooker. Procurement in cold blood was not his style. And the cost of contracting an STD — the mercury cure being almost as painful as pleasure's plague itself — made the whore a desperate measure.

The Casanovan should seriously consider the lesser of two venereal evils. Fly solo. [*See* ONANISM]

～ Heartbreak

"I went back to my room, careless of the future, broken down by the deepest of sorrows. I locked myself in and went to bed. I was in a state of complete moral and physical apathy."

Yes, even the most swinging of swains is vulnerable to the heartbreak of a ruptured romance. The circumstances of being swamped by sorrow may vary — the lady decides to go back to her husband/ her day job/ her home in a place off the local bus route. The effect is the same: utter desolation.

The victim may, like Giacomo, take to his bed, in a darkened room, and refuse to eat more than three meals a day. If required to go to the workplace to spare the family the funeral expenses after he sucks the gas pipe, his fellow employees find him moody, unable to concentrate on his *Playboy* calendar.

The Casanovan who believes himself to be immune to heartbreak, because his whole dogma of relationships with women is based on freedom from commitment, is in for a rude shock. From time to time he will become emotionally involved with a pretty and clever girl who sees him for what he is (a butterfly), enjoys him for the flutter, pins him to her collection, and moves on to a specimen more substantial.

Does if help that we recognize that what has been wounded so grievously is our ego? Not a whit. Also futile: telling ourself (as we lie there morosely chewing our pillow): "Hey, she's not the only pebble on the beach." We didn't buy those Reeboks to impress riprap.

The only solace: assure ourself that any woman who passes up the opportunity to do what we want is clearly mentally unstable. She may *appear* to be quite rational, enough so to drive us crazy. But the defective gene is in there somewhere, and the upside of our misery is that we have avoided parenting a defective child. Probably a son who turns out to be a cross-dresser.

Whatever the therapy, sooner or later, like Giacomo, the Casanovan will recover from his heartbreak. It is not one of the life-threatening cardiac conditions. And it bears testament to his being, after all, only human.

❧ Hips

"My lovely Frenchwoman wore a blue coat which did not conceal her attractive person and in order to ascertain, even at first sight, that she was not a man, it was sufficient to look at her hips. She was too well made as a woman ever to pass for a man."

The hips are a clear giveaway. Even the girl clad and padded as goalie for Canada's female ice hockey team has hips that remove any suspicion that she is Gump Worsley, trying to make a comeback.

Casanova read women's hips well. Although much of his attention was directed towards BREASTS, ample hips were the main indication of gender below the waist. (Along with small FEET.)

He understood that the hips can be more believable than any other means of feminine communication. Including the eyes and mouth. A woman's hips will contradict what is being said by expressions more directly controlled by the mind. They live a salacious life of their own. Perhaps because they are relatively distant from the brain, hips are noteworthy.

Casanova understood hip talk. (Which has nothing to do with our contemporary jargon of the pubescent.) For instance, he comprehended nothing of the Spanish language till he danced the fandango with a lady of Spain whose hips transcended the language barrier.

What a woman does with her hips — cocking and aiming — predicts of course how lithely sensational she will be during intercourse. The old joke — "Are you sexually active?" "No, I just lie there." — reflects something of how the hips may serve merely as support for a belt.

The ultimate message of a woman's hips: here lies the purlieu of the pelvic basin, set to cradle the unborn. Woe to the Casanovan who ignores the purpose that goes beyond the invitation!

The sobering fact is that the parts of a woman's anatomy exciting the male most are those planted by Mother Nature to generate more of the species. So, hooray for hips! But remember: they are loaded for bearing.

Honesty

The man who deliberately deceives a woman to get sex is not worthy of the title of Casanovan. He is a cad. He may be a very satisfied cad, but he belongs to a lower order of lover, frequenting a moral sewer.

If there *is* a Hell, he is bound for the barbie.

What of the man who deceives himself, about what he feels for a woman? This lad believes his own professions of undying love, failing to understand that most loves have a mortality rate that makes them uninsurable.

Casanova, however, made no claims for his love except that fulfilling it with a woman was the most important thing in his life. At the moment. He was totally honest. He documents himself to the lovely Thérèse:

"You suppose me wealthy, and I am not so; as soon as what is now in my purse is spent I shall have nothing left. You may fancy that I was born a patrician, but my social condition is really inferior to your own. I have no lucrative talents, no profession, nothing to give me the assurance that I am able to earn my living. I have neither relatives nor friends, nor claims upon anyone, and I have no serious plan or purpose before me. All I possess is youth, health, courage, some intelligence, honour, honesty, and some tincture of letters . . . With all that, I am naturally inclined to extravagance. Lovely Thérèse, you have my portrait. What is your answer?"

Well, what woman could say nay?

Given such a titillating display of naked truth, only she with a hidden agenda would fail to succumb.

Honesty may be the most powerful aphrodisiac a man can depend on, to sway the feminine fancy. Liquor, as poet Ogden Nash said, is quicker, but honesty has the appeal of being both non-conventional and kinder to the liver.

After all, of what avail to a Casanovan, to contrive to cohabit with a woman if he can't live with himself?

Casanova, the consummate gambler, with a woman, put all his cards on the table — and rarely lost. Never did he waste energy and time plotting ploys in the game of love. With this man, what a woman saw was what she got. And by his accounts, at least, honesty was not only the best policy, it was insurance beyond the wildest dreams of Allstate.

❧ Horoscopes

How to persuade a young woman to leave the family home and accompany you to another town, where her natural impulses will be less constrained by parental guidance? It's a problem that can occur from time to time, for the light-footed libertine dedicated to letting no grass grow under his feet when making hay.

Casanova's technique: make the distant field look greener:

". . . I cast the horoscope for Mlle. Anne. As I hoped to take her to Paris with me, I predicted that she would become "her master's mistress," i.e. the king's consort and mother of a royal prince. To spur a quick decision, the prophecy warned that "the king would need to see her before her eighteenth birthday . . ." Or her fate would turn to mush.

In this instance, the quarry refused the bait. Mlle. Anne balked at bounding into bed with the prophet, as a reward for his getting her a promotion to Mrs. Louis XV. Casanova saw that marriage was the only means of gratifying his desire for this luscious homebody, a stark and awful prospect: ". . . my obsessive fear of losing my freedom won." And he decamped for Paris. Solo.

After a brief eclipse by Rationalism, daily horoscopes are once again very influential with young women, often taking up whole pages in the tacky tabloid. Yet the Casanovan may profit from their prophecies, and exploit the Zodiac to persuade a young woman that her good fortune does indeed lie in a weekend for two at Whistler.

Whereas it is bad form to deliberately deceive a member of the fair sex, the credulity of women is a hidden asset for the Casanovan, perhaps the only advantage he has against their superior cunning.

On the other hand, if he reads his own horoscope and is told that this is the day when he will meet the person of his dreams, he should check the expiry date on his bottle of reality pills.

⮞ Horticulture

Aside from sowing his wild oats, Casanova shows perfunctory interest in other types of agriculture. Paraphrasing Pope, he would have said that the proper study of mankind is woman.

It was to further this study that Casanova followed the fair maid Barberine into her family's garden to pick figs from their one tree . . .

"I held the ladder while she climbed up to look. I looked too."

"'My dear Barberine, what do you think I can see?'"

"'What you have often seen with my sister.'"

"'True! But you are prettier than she.'"

"She did not reply, but placed her foot on a high branch and showed me a most seductive picture. I was in ecstasy. Barberine, seeing it, did not hurry to move. When I helped her to descend, my hand wandered indiscreetly, and I asked her if the fruit had been plucked. She took her time to assure me that it was quite fresh."

"'Will you give me what I have apprehended, my dear?'"

"'My mother is going to Muran tomorrow, where she will stay for the day. If you come to me, there is nothing I shall deny you . . .'"

Evidently, Casanova had a green thumb, plus four other fecund digits.

So, does this mean that the Casanovan should include ladder climbing in his repertoire of effective groping? Yes, certainly, if he can work it into his fitness program. [*See* LADDERS]

It would perhaps be a mistake, however, to hang around fig-tree orchards, hoping to catch a befrocked lass in the act of ascending a ladder and obviously in need of a boost.

Probably the more promising area of horticulture for the Casanovan hoping to fondle something is the produce section of his local supermarket. He will be competing (usually) with fewer flies, bees and birds, and, with practice, will learn to squeeze fruit with a cunning hand that arouses other, female shoppers. What Jacques could have done, reaching for the same melon with a gorgeous matron!

Leave the tree to Eve.

⮞ Humbug

Casanova always made it clear to a woman that sharing her thoughts was not his entire interest in her.

No humbug in this man's approach. His first gaze not only undressed a woman with his eyes but carried her part of the distance to the nearest bed.

Here the Casanovan should note that, for a woman, the difference between being eyed (good) and being ogled (bad) depends largely on the height and other physical features of the viewer. Short, fat, ugly guys leer. The tall Adonis regards admiringly.

Now, what about his getting humbug from a *woman*? This can be much harder to detect, because a woman uses her whole body to create humbug, whereas a man just uses his mouth and maybe a sincere necktie.

Just by making a project of crossing her legs — especially if wearing fishnet nylons — a woman can give a man ideas that turn out to be a very expensive type of humbug, one that leaves him lying on a stretcher in Emergency with his nose in a sling.

A sampling of situations in which the Casanovan should suspect that he is being made the victim of humbuggery:

1. Your girl friend blames her chin's bad case of beard burn on eating prickly pear.
2. The sweater she says she knitted for you bears the label Made in Afghanistan.
3. Your fiancée tells you "I love you, John" when your name is Fred.
4. The girl you first dated in April tells you in May you have to get married in June because she's six months pregnant.

~ Husbands

As a devout Casanovan, what is your ritual when, having had sex with a woman, you meet her years later in the company of her husband? Especially if she flies into your arms and kisses you ardently?

It is easy to become flummoxed by this situation, especially if the husband is unusually large, with smoked hams for hands. But not Casanova. Because of his remarkable number of affairs, in many different cities, it was a common occurrence for him to have to explain, extempore, why some husband's wife was hanging around his neck, and ogling him for auld lang syne.

As a rule the wife assumes damage control. Thérèse, for instance, tells hubby:

"My dear, you see before you my father."

On cue, Casanova confirms: "Yes, sir, your Thérèse is my daughter, my sister, my cherished friend. She is an angel, and this treasure is your wife."

"Yes, I know," says the thoroughly confused husband.

Casanova then embraces the husband, whom Thérèse asks to make some chocolate for their guest. While the husband is busy in the kitchen, Thérèse again rushes into Casanova's arms . . .

"Tomorrow we will be like brother and sister. Today let us be lovers."

Nothing loath, Casanova accedes: ". . . Our transports were mutual and we renewed them again and again during the half hour the chocolate was being made . . ."

Now, Jacques was extremely fond of his CHOCOLATE. The scene above gives us an inkling why. The Casanovan does not enjoy the same advantage, today, a nice cup of cocoa being quicker to prepare, thus keeping a hubby less occupied in the kitchen.

Later in the same visit to town, Casanova meets Thérèse's son, whom he recognizes immediately as *his* son too. Thérèse introduces the boy as her brother, thus compounding the confusion of relationships. Left alone with Casanova, Thérèse asks him if he would care to give his son a brother. As this would put a strain on the supply of chocolate, Casanova declines, with thanks and an early departure from town.

The point is, if he has had a truly fulfilling (for both) affair with a woman, the Casanovan has nothing to fear from meeting her with her husband. She will cover for him. Gladly. Wives remember ex-lovers more fondly than the man they are married to. The familiar breeds contempt, whereas the unattainable remains ever lovely.

[Note: some medical scientists believe that chocolate may be bad for the prostate. But then most good things are.]

✒ Hypocrisy

Did Casanova really believe that his memoirs would become a handbook for parents of daughters? A lay bible? Or an emergency manual of instructions to be kept handy, like what to do in the event of an earthquake?

The warning that he may have had in mind, for parents, was to watch out for sex maniacs with no other qualifications, as tenured lovers. Note that he mentions his paying "homage." There can be no doubt that he regarded every beautiful woman as an earthly goddess, whom he worshipped in the only ways he knew how: on his knees, on his back, and just about every other devotional position available to the human body.

Casanova paid homage to women on the installment plan. For life.

Hypocrisy, says La Rochefoucauld, "is the homage that vice pays to virtue." But today virtue has no fixed address. Recently in the States, a female school teacher was arrested and jailed for having sex with one of her male students, a minor. One dares say that many other highschool lads now look forward to being sexually perverted by their attractive teacher. They may actually seek a detention, after class, in hopes of losing their virginity in an academic setting. Sex on a desk can be hard on the back, but nobody said that learning is easy.

In this social environment of egalitarian perversion, the Casanovan has less need to play the hypocrite in his memoirs.

Besides, today there is no market for a book detailing the sexual exploits of a man. Women authors have taken over the conjugately explicit. And fathers and mothers get all the warnings they need from *Consumer Reports.*

⧟ Identification

"They all look alike in the dark." This crass platitude Casanova never accepted, yet he still managed to get himself into awkward situations that might have been avoided with better lighting.

Instance: the evening when he accepts a ride home in the carriage of the Count de la Tour d'Auvergne, who is accompanied by that gentleman's lady friend. Never able to resist the presence of a pretty woman, Casanova takes advantage of the compressed company and darkness to take a dainty hand and cover it with silent kisses. He then hears the count remark:

"I am much obliged to you, dear sir, for an attention totally Italian, but of which I do not feel worthy." Casanova hastily aborts his groping at a wrong sleeve, and must endure peals of laughter to which he adds his own, good sport that he hates to be.

A much more mortifying episode involved Casanova's midnight rendezvous with a gorgeous guest in his house, in which also roomed an ugly witch whom he had offended. As he waits in his bed and darkness, his hand is grasped and he is guided to a sofa, where he "renews again and again the pledges of my ardent love," then retreats ere it be dawn. The next morning he encounters his dream girl looking peeved about having waited in bed for him all night. "What unforeseen accident prevented your coming?"

Giacomo has, of course, come, again and again, but to the wrong terminus: the witch who has the last cackle, and writes him mocking letters. Casanova is so devastated that he closes the house and moves to another town.

Thanks to Thomas Edison, the Casanovan is at less hazard to duplicate the circumstances of mistaken identity that blemished the maestro's record. Unless he goes camping, that is. In mixed company. Also, over-consumption of alcohol can induce a loss of visual acuity that gets a man into the wrong sleeping bag.

Another ID problem: in the darkened cinema, seated beside an unidentified female, you feel a warm pressure against your knee. What should you do? Answer: leave the movie house at once and wait for the video.

☞ Impotence

Rarely did Casanova have difficulty in rising to the occasion. The two mortifying episodes that he recounts — with customary respect for the unflattering fact — were temporary, the result of, so to speak, flooding his carburetor . . .

". . . I was in a frenzy of rage. I had never had such a misfortune, unless as the result of complete exhaustion, or from a strong mental impression capable of destroying my natural faculties. Let my readers imagine what I suffered in the flower of my age, with a strong constitution, holding the body of a woman I had ardently desired in my arms, while she tenderly caressed me, and yet I could do nothing for her. I was in despair; one cannot offer a greater insult to a woman."

A tragedy. Euripides wrote no drama more affecting. Our hero has taken a mortal blow to his self-esteem. Well, maybe not mortal. But it certainly ruined his day.

How could such a disaster strike our icon in the one area — the Achilles heel gone north a bit — where he seemed invulnerable? Answer: he has spent all of the previous night doing strenuous battle with two sisters, Annette and Véronique, a contest involving more amatory combinations and permutations than the game plan of the San Francisco Forty-niners.

Could this happen to the Casanovan? Probably not, today's sisters being less likely to copulate as a combo. But he is even more susceptible to the cause of impotence cited by Casanova: mental distraction. It is absolutely vital: the ability to maintain focus on the task at hand. To concentrate, without grinding the teeth. To clear the mind of other concerns, such as what is happening to one's mutual fund.

What should be going up is fatally compromised by what is going down.

Thanks to Casanova's exemplary freedom from extraneous thoughts while making love, real impotence did not strike him till he reached sixty. Then he sat down to chronicle the many, many times he had avoided insulting a woman, usually by a wide margin.

We must be truly grateful that this normally indefatigable lover did not have access to modern sex potions like Viagra. The priceless memoirs might never have been written, and succeeding generations of men would have lost the gospel according to Jacques.

∽ Incest

The scenario: while holidaying abroad you, the Casanovan, encounter an old flame, whose attractive young daughter — *your* daughter — is married to a wealthy older man who has delusions of achieving paternity. The mother, who wants a grandchild, not on with her elderly son-in-law, sets you up with her daughter, who nine months later gives birth to a son. The boy gives you the distinction of being both the father and the grandfather of the same child. Would this make your day?

Even Casanova was unsettled by this incestuous episode. The only thing that made him feel better about it was that, some years later, on meeting his double progeny grown to a young man, he saw a resemblance to the dad rather than the father. A victory of nurture over nature, for which Casanova was extremely grateful. As an old man he was able to welcome the invitation to his son's/grandson's wedding, with a conscience if not clear at least somewhat less clouded.

The Casanovan is not apt to experience the situation that invites incest. Just as well, since this form of sexual activity is one of the few that still raise eyebrows, if not the possibility of a sojourn in a correctional facility.

There are still some no-nos out there, Elmer.

❧ Income

Casanova had no steady income. He also had no steady girlfriend. He was unsteady on all accounts. As an Italian, his financial structure was modeled on the Leaning Tower of Pisa.

Was this a disadvantage for him, in attracting women? Not unless he wanted to be trampled by the herd. Casanova proved, definitively, that while earning a steady income, with a comfortable financial future, may help to win a man a wife, it is irrelevant to a man in command of his senses.

So long as the Casanovan is generous — indeed, profligate — in his spending his money to entertain his lady, she will not quibble about those of his resources that are not warm to the touch.

For Casanova, his income was funded by one asset: his personal charm. This mother lode was so rich that, years after he last made love to her, an old sweetheart would ship him some cash to cover his hotel bill.

Casanova supplemented his allowance from Mme d'Urfé, the mad moneybag of Paris, by gambling. He learned early on what we all know to be true today: the banker can't lose. So long as he had the physical stamina to keep the faro game going for a matter of days, eventually the law of averages would rule in his favour.

Does this mean that the Casanovan should give up that soul-destroying job at the post-office, and depend entirely on winning the Lotto? Obviously not. What it does mean is that he may have to choose between playing golf (the most costly and cruel mistress that a man can embrace) and showing a girl a really good time.

Owning flashy, top-of-the-line skis butters no parsnips if he hasn't money left to lavish on Ms. Snow Bunny.

Giacomo, whose animal magnetism was strong enough to alter the orbits of heavenly bodies, knew that it is folly to expect a woman to be grateful for sex without the trimmings.

So, the Casanovan must understand that, regardless of the source and size of his income, he should be prudent enough to focus his major expenditure on one objective: women. The marvelous saving bond that will enrich his old age with memories.

ᵛ Infatuation

Infatuation may be defined as sexual LOVE as experienced by someone else. Usually someone younger than we are. Often a member of our immediate family. Our teenage children become infatuated with older teenage children, and the condition may persist well into middle age.

Romeo and Juliet suffered from infatuation. In fact it killed them, eventually, though Shakespeare does manage to make the crush sound serious.

Casanova too had bouts of infatuation. The first when he was about twelve and a boarder in the home of his mentor, the young priest Dr. Gozzi. Casanova got bathed every morning by Dr. Gozzi's thirteen-year-old sister, Bettina — "pretty, lively, a great reader of romance." One morning, while washing his legs, she "carried her love for cleanliness too far," causing him "such intense voluptuousness that it did not stop till it could go no farther."

Bingo. Infatuation with an older woman.

Unfortunately, Bettina already had a lover. "When I caught the clod coming out of Bettina's room early one morning, he gave me a furious kick in the stomach which I believed cured me of my infatuation." The unheroic measure.

If infatuation is ADORATION with a fillip of folly, how then can the Casanovan tell whether his fondness is sensible or he is just ga-ga about the girl? As the song goes: is it the real turtle soup, or only the mock?

Not easy. The French have a relevant saying: in every love affair there is the one who loves and the one who allows himself to love. Clearly, it is safer to be the party of the second part, more in control of his dementia.

Sometimes the smitten Casanovan can usefully ask a trusted old friend — assuming that he has one — for an opinion on the probability of his being merely infatuated with this woman who has him plucking the coverlet, sleepless with concern about his choice of after-shave.

At the very least, he should avoid letting her wash his legs in bed. Some women have an idle curiosity about a man's physical response to being laundered. This should never be confused with true devotion.

~ Infidelity

Never being married, Casanova had no serious problem with infidelity. He puts his own spin on the sin. E.g., when he encounters a pair of pussycats with whom he has played (ensemble) in the past, he is tempted to cheat only on his current squeeze: "I could see the eyes of my dear little wives sparkling with devilish anticipation, and they reconquered all their influence over my heart, in spite of my love for Thérèse, whose image was, all the same, brilliant in my soul. *This was passing infidelity, but not inconstancy.*" (Ed's italics)

Such was Giacomo's creed of faithfulness. He could do nothing about his being wildly attracted to other women — especially those he had engaged in unholy matrimony. But he remained constant to his woman of the hour.

The Casanovan — also, by definition, not married in the conventional sense of the word — will do well to emulate the Master. That is, do not start a love affair till the previous affair is over for both parties. (This never happens, of course. One party is nearly always the dumper, the other the dumpee, so that acceptance is complete only for the former. But the theory is sound.)

Even though this personal religion requires that he remain single, there is one person to whom the Casanovan must remain true: himself. "I'm always true to you, darling, in my fashion" makes a fun pop song lyric, but a lousy lifestyle. Okay, so she is only his "significant other." Making fidelity pretty damn fuzzy. Still, she should have all of him, so long as he has enough of her.

ᕦᕤ Intellect

"When intellect enters on the field, the heart has to yield." A memorable bit of quasi-verse, from our lover reflecting on his matching minds with the many-faceted Clementine.

The beautiful woman who supplements her superior instincts with a formidable intellect can scare the id right out of a guy. At least temporarily. He becomes so involved in heady discussion, in the passion of debate, that he forgets what he had in mind when he rented the canoe.

"I was astonished to find that during all the hours we had spent together she had not caused the slightest sexual feeling to arise in me . . ." (Give that lady a cigar!) Wha hoppen? "It was certainly not virtue, for I do not carry virtue so far as that. Then what was it? . . . The fine things we read together interested us so strongly that we did not think of love . . ."

Ah-ha! BOOKS. Beware of women bearing books! Especially feminist books. Many of these treacherous tomes are paperbacks. Easily concealed in a belly pouch. Or in the overnight bag that the Casanovan fondly imagines to contain nothing but black-lace lingerie and handcuffs.

"Let me not to the marriage of true minds admit impediments . . ." But Shakespeare was a bit of a dreamer. For the Casanovan in the 21st century, getting wedded in his mind may land him in the sand-trap. Concentration is indivisible.

Yet Casanova was able to overcome the temporary IMPOTENCE

imposed by Clementine's mesmeric intellect, and did bed her bookless. And it turned out to be one of his most unforgettable affairs, and durable friendships. If the Casanovan has a well-muscled patience — exercised by playing chess or fishing for steelhead — he too may achieve the ideal union of both physical and mental qualities.

The main thing is: don't be overawed by a woman's intellect to the point of assuming that she could never be interested in a guy who thinks that PBS is a women's condition.

A woman too — even the brainiest — can be a sucker for a great set of buns. She will be happy to conform to whatever intellect the Casanovan has, so long as he shows a willingness to learn and doesn't drool in public.

As Giacomo demonstrated to Clementine, reciprocity of knowledge is one of the glories of a human relationship. We should all be so lucky.

⌁ Intuition

"The instinct of women teaches them greater secrets than all the philosophy and the research of men."

So sayeth Casanova, speaking as an older if not wiser man.

He was, of course, bang-on. Female intuition is the most formidable weapon in the sex's armoury, more than compensating for a woman's sometimes having the IQ of a gerbil.

A woman can know what a man is going to do before *he* does — often by a matter of days. She intuits it. Why, then, does a woman often get into trouble with Mr. Wrong? Ans: because she lets her intuition be overruled by reason — that error-prone mechanism of the mind.

In computer terms, women's intuition is the hardware, men's logic the floppy disc.

How, then, did Casanova manage to score so many seductions against an inscrutable force? The male's only ally against a woman's intuition is her vanity, in believing that she is armed with so many charms that a man must succumb to COMMITMENT. The ease with which Jacques was bewitched by those physical features, their effect clearly visible even in bad light, convinced his target that she could ignore her instincts as a false alarm. By the time she realized that Casanova's passionate impulses were no match for his even stronger desire to remain single, he had hit the road.

Has female intuition been dulled by the feminism that encourages a woman to think like a man? Was that sixth, or seventh, sense more sharply honed when a woman's whole existence, her making her way in the world, depended on her intuitive appraisal of a man as Mr. Right?

Probably. No one, not even Oprah, can be good at everything.

However, the Casanovan will find it prudent to assume nothing about the role of intuition in his rejection. Consider that today's mature woman has had a wider, and deeper, experience of men than the fifteen-year-old virgins whose instincts fought a losing battle with Casanova's libidinous mettle.

Accept it, man: you are, by nature, instinctually disadvantaged. Proceed with caution.

❧ Italian

Does the Casanova disciple need to be Italian, to succeed as a great lover? Ans: No, but it helps. Certainly more than just being double-jointed.

Who is it that ranks as the undisputed icon of ADORATION by North American women? Frank Sinatra, of course. A skinny crooner with the morals of a mink, Sinatra nevertheless has had millions of women lusting for him despite all the flat notes he ululated.

Old Blue Eyes had the Italian Boldness that made him, for women, a one-man Mafia — to kill for.

Sinatra and Casanova. Jacques too was fully aware of the advantage he enjoyed, as a lover, in having the genetic background of the Boot. To be an Italian made him, he knew, cock of the wooer's walk. Thus when momentarily stalled in his advances upon a beautiful young actress whose alleged maidenhood had withstood assault by other panting swains, Casanova notes:

"I was merely amused, for her former lovers had been French-men, more accomplished in assault than in triumphing over the artful dodges of a girl. I was an Italian, and knew everything required, so I never doubted my victory."

Having proved his point, and found that her maidenhood was a work of fiction, he "rewarded her as if I had been the first to bite the cherry."

This is the sort of sexual self-assurance that brings millions of anglicized female tourists to Italy, every year, for the purported purpose of viewing the ceiling of the Sistine Chapel. And, less explicitly, other wonders best admired from the supine position.

The Italian mystique. Thus when Shakespeare, an Englishman, needs a romantic hero for his tragedy of love conquering all, whom does he choose? Romeo, of course. Not Fred, or Ludwig, or even Pierre. Only an ardent son of Verona could credibly breathe to the balconied Juliet "O! that I were a glove upon that hand, that I might touch that cheek . . ." When the current Prince Charles is overheard saying to his aging Camilla: "I wish I could be your tampon," he demonstrates why English males have been more successful in establishing representative government than in romancing English women.

However, no man should blame his lack of success with the other sex on his not being descended from the conquering Caesar. Race should not be used as a crutch, except in parts of northern Ontario. Just select a really nice Chianti, for your dinner date, and think positivo.

⁓ Jealousy

Casanova was rarely victimized by the green-eyed monster. He was such a charmer that once a woman had been taken with his over-whelming sex appeal, no rival stood a ghost of a chance. Jealousy was something he created in other men, the poor stiffs who had to stand by and watch as women they desired bowed to the conqueror like wildflowers to a prevailing wind.

However, the one time when Casanova did become jealous, he really made a meal of it. After several nights of amorous delight with the fair Thérèse, he is stricken with the pending arrival in town of her fiancé . . .

". . . to have only just lifted the nectar to my lips, and to see the precious cup escape my hands! I was in a fearful state of perplexity. I could not make up my mind to consent to her marrying, nor could I resolve to wed her myself . . ."

The classic quandary! Gored by the horns of the dilemma, who of us has not known this agony? (Okay, you can put down your hands now.)

When Thérèse — with the damnable reasonableness of woman — asks Giacomo to tell her whether she should marry her fiancé, he replies that she should do so if she likes the guy that much.

"From that moment she refused to give me even one final embrace." Cruel, cruel! "I was now assailed with most anguished remorse and jealousy." Distraught, Casanova charges over to his rival's lodging, determined to kill him in a duel or, failing response to that challenge, just "assassinate him."

Luckily the groom-to-be greets him as a friend of the family and is so generally pleasant that the jilted lover is restored to a semblance of sanity.

Casanova had, however, come within a hair of getting himself hanged for murder — which would have put a definite crimp in his career as the world's greatest lover.

The message: the Casanovan may save himself a deal of misery if he checks his date's left hand for the engagement ring. The bigger the diamond, the larger the headache if he becomes emotionally involved with a woman who has the ace up her sleeve.

Her wedding ring, however, does not imply the same potential for being made jealous. That woman has her security, and is merely diverting herself with a once-in-a-lifetime opportunity. It is misguided of the Casanovan to become jealous of a woman's husband — that prisoner of matrimony.

Fear the rivalry of the wolf in the wild, not in the zoo's cage.

ᕦ Judgment

"I had long been accustomed to reading women's characters by the play of their features, and the physiognomy of my charmer declared her to be a lover of pleasure."

Casanova here is telling how, while pondering a career change from libertine/ adventurer to taker of holy orders, he happened to be gazing out his window when "an elegant lady" stepped from her carriage below and responded to his gaze — that telepathic power that women have — with a long look that eliminated the possibility of his mounting the pulpit, instead.

Casanova's ability to judge a woman's potential for sensational sex was infallible, for distances up to a hundred yards. In fog.

This is one of those skills that cannot be learned. Experience helps, of course, but unless the Casanovan has the instinctive, and immediate, response to the "physiognomy" of a woman, he must depend on directives from authoritative texts, such as the *Sports Illustrated* swimsuit edition.

Fortunately, most heterosexual men in reasonable health, and with sight in at least one eye, will share something of Jacques' 20/20 reading of the woman hot to trot. Marilyn Monroe, for example, impacted instantly on every male human in the known universe. The hooded, bedroom eyes, the mouth writhing in a plea for sexual satiety, could draw a whimper from a brass Buddha.

Marilyn was a victim of her own voluptuousness, as were many of the women on whom Casanova zeroed in with unerring accuracy. He was the Cruise missile of pleasure-seeking men.

However, the Cupid's-bow lips and dimpled chin may bespeak a mind that loses its balance when the body assumes the vertical position. This can impair a relationship of any duration longer than a summer's night. Helen of Troy had the face that launched a thousand ships, and a war that benefitted only the wooden-horse industry. Which proved that beauty alone can be hazardous to your health.

The Casanovan should also be aware that the sensuality he recognizes in a woman's features is not apt to be a unique discovery, such as Banting's synthesizing insulin. Other men are just as perceptive, if not more so, with the result that escorting a sexpot in public can expose you to collateral damage, the radiation from toxic gazes.

But one should not shrink from the challenge. Only as a last resort should the Casanovan settle for the sensible-looking woman with no overt interest in immoderate sex. After Marilyn, President Kennedy still had Jackie. And died with no cause for regret.

Keepsakes

"I cut off a tuft of her fleece and a lock of her beautiful hair, promising her always to wear them next to my heart . . . Next morning I was on the road to Chambéry."

As a travelling man, Casanova has frequent occasion to take a keepsake, an intimate memento, of the woman he has ravished. Just a sentimental fool? Not at all. This lover was enough of a gentleman to give his conquest reason to believe that the sexual episode has been, for him at least, memorable. It's a touch of class.

It is sometimes impossible to avoid the tears — not to mention, in some cases, a hurled bedroom clock — that accompany breakup. But this painful scene can be mitigated by an exchange of souvenirs. Of which Casanova always seemed to have an ample supply. Often these were portraits of himself. He knew, perhaps instinctively, that he might well run into the woman again, on his next circuit of the Continent. And his having a friend in court could depend on his having had a friend in bed.

It was to expedite the exchange of keepsakes that Jacques took "a tuft of fleece" and lock of cranial hair — surely the most touching depilatory on record. It certainly preempted the sort of rotten barbering job that Delilah inflicted on Samson.

Whether or not the Casanovan chooses to replay the rape of the lock, upper and lower, he should perhaps hesitate to promise always to wear this keepsake next to his heart. Over time, and especially if he already has a hairy chest, this pledge may become excessively hirsute. Yet a promise made in the knowledge that it cannot be kept is a violation of the Casanovan code of honour. All your body hair may fall off. None of it cherished by anyone else.

∽ Keyholes

"I watched through the key-hole, and saw the two sisters come into the room . . . Then my two beauties, their door once locked, sat down on the sofa and completed their night toilet, which in that fortunate climate is similar to the costume of our first mother . . . exposing most secret beauties to my profane eyes . . . "

"Happy moments which I can no longer enjoy, but the sweet remembrance of which death alone can make me lose!"

Thus, the aging Casanova's touching tribute to the simple joy provided him, as a lad, by the keyhole. The voyeur's best and oldest friend.

So much simpler to operate than telescope or binoculars — one's hands do tremble, right? — is this ready aperture. Also, the perfect means for a woman to deliberately display herself — stripping provocatively down to bare naked — knowing that she is being watched, but without the overt exhibitionism of Macy's window.

It is a grievous loss: they don't make keyholes the way they did in Jacques' time. Keys then were enormous, and their holes accordingly large enough to afford even the most bugged eye a full range of viewing. Today, most inside doors have no keyhole at all. They lock with a button or, if security is really tight, an electronic device that identifies the eyeball as that of an accredited peeping Tom.

Deprived of the bedroom keyhole, the Casanovan has little opportunity to enjoy private peeping without having to crawl through the air-conditioning system — a claustrophobic exercise, and apt to be too noisy to be ignored by even the most cooperative occupant.

Yes, Casanova did enjoy certain technological advantages, lost to the millennial eye. Including that device for sighting celestial bodies: the keyhole.

⇜ Kisses

"Kisses — that mute, yet expressive language, that delicate, voluptuous contact which sends sentiment coursing rapidly through the veins, which expresses at the same time the feeling of the heart and the impressions of the mind . . ." Casanova's sensitive definition of *kissing*.

The more prosaic: uptown shopping for downtown goods.

Whichever we accept, on the evidence Casanova was a kisser *sans pareil*. Once a woman had given him her lips, the rest of her body was as good as conceded. Only very occasionally did he encounter a beautiful and desirable woman (Esther), whose discretion was so iron-clad that it defied the natural progression from bussing to bedding . . .

"She was lavish of nothing but her kisses, but kisses are rather irritating than soothing."

Our man refers here to kisses that are perfunctory pecks, rather than the abandoned type of labial conjunction. Some women are free with these inconclusive kisses, and hugs, used as a way of thanking a man for some service other than the one he aimed to provide.

Casanova never goes into clinical detail, regarding his kissing technique. We might, for instance, expect that a philanderer who spent so many profitable years in France would expatiate on the French kiss, for the enlightenment of future generations. A pity, this, because many Casanovans have little guide but what they observe in sexy films, with no idea what to do with their tongue once the mouth is open for business.

What we see, in these pornish flicks, is two (or more) persons who seem to be making a meal of each other's face.

These are the kisses of a couple in a hurry lest their cell phone should claim attention.

The Casanovan may, therefore, be surprised to find how effective it can be to kiss a lady's hand — the fingers first, then, if all goes well, her palm. Then, northward, ho!

Or, if a kiss is to be the goal of an intimate dinner for two, their sucking on the opposite ends of a strand of spaghetti can help to prepare her for the inevitable.

But kissing is one social skill that cannot be taught. The Casanovan must learn through trial and error, always remembering that the toothless smile is a high price to pay for his mistake.

~ Lactation

"I shall have to call you 'baby,'" says one of Jacques' adorable nuns, after giving birth to a child which — for a change — was not fathered by the venereal Venetian.

What prompts this informal christening is the occasion of Casanova's kissing the new mother's bountiful breast and finding nourishment for more than the soul.

"It is very sweet, my darling, and the small drop I tasted made me so happy. You will not be angry at me relishing this innocent privilege."

The nun assures him that he is a worthy surrogate for the neonate that has been hustled off to an orphanage.

Most Casanovans will not have the opportunity to enjoy the experience of tasting post-natal drip. Today's nun is more likely to retain the child and forego the pope, a loss to both orphanages and lads who like their loving *au lait*.

But it was so typical of Casanova that no sensual experience was too earthy for him to enjoy. In our era of bottle-fed babies, men tend to forget that the female breast is a functional part of women's anatomy, with a purpose other than to nurture a bikini bra.

Casanova appreciated this noble structure [*see* BREASTS] for its beauty, but did not shrink from the reality of its role in human reproduction. Certainly he would never understand "Baby" as the favourite sobriquet in our *chansons d'amour* — ambisexual and smacking of infantilism. One name fits all — loosely.

The thinking Casanovan will eschew the "baby" talk, when addressing his sweetheart, even though it means having to remember her name. How he feels, personally, about the benefits of breast-feeding probably depends on how addicted he is to sucking his thumb. Certainly an interesting source of calcium.

➤ Ladders

Aptitude with ladders should be part of the Casanovan's amatory job description. The master himself had recourse to this means of informal ascent, several times, though not always in order to access a woman situated above ground level. His celebrated roof-top escape from The Leads prison, for example, and other jail breaks, made him familiar with the ladder to the extent of qualifying as a fireman, had he not preferred to work solo.

Like Romeo's ascension unto Juliet on an upper-floor balcony, Casanova's use of the ladder was to bypass persons in the building who might impede his progress with a lady. Such as the lay-sister charged with the security of the beautiful nun whom he had spotted during a stop-over in Aix-les-Bains, and whom he thought he recognized as an earlier conquest.

Having tailed her to her house, and been alerted that his nun is guarded by the vestal watchdog, Casanova enlists the cottage owner . . .

". . . The peasant woman helped me ascend to my dear Marie-Madeleine's window by a ladder . . . I covered the nun's adorable face with ardent kisses . . ."

Well, it turns out that the nun is not his dear Marie-Madeleine, but Casanova adjusts readily to mistaken identity, and soon becomes the lover of Marie-Madeleine Mark II. (We wonder at Casanova's proclivity for sisters to whom he was not related except by sex. The temptation is to call him a nun's habit. It must be resisted.)

But what woman, sororal or not, could resist the man risking life and limb to climb an unfamiliar ladder, in the dark, to reach her room? Comparatively, ascension by the building elevator, or even climbing several flights of stairs, count as much less of a dramatic, obstacle-surmounting feat. Yawnsville, in fact.

It is common knowledge that one reason why women lust for firemen is this willingness to take heroic measures, if only to put out a fire. Therefore the Casanovan should seize any opportunity to climb a ladder for a lady, even if only to clean her roof gutters. (Check first that her home insurance covers personal injury.)

ᴝ Language

"I might have had her, then and there, for ten guineas. I did not care to do so, however, for though charming she could speak only English, and I liked to have all my senses, including hearing, gratified."

Casanova fussy? Perhaps. But a case can be made for understanding what your lover is saying. Especially during intercourse, when women have been known to talk. The Casanovan may assume that hearing may be sacrificed to other senses — sight, smell, touch and (optional) taste.

Our connoisseur is more demanding.

Also, Casanova would have found English a particularly asexual language in which to engage in pillow talk. Despite some gentling by the introduction of French words after the Norman Conquest, English lacks the sensual tones of the Romance tongue. The very word love — often neutered to "luv" or, worse, "loov" — is no match for the sexy sound of *l'amour . . . amore.*

Thus Casanova made love in French almost exclusively, with Italian and Spanish as second choices. His affairs in German were, predictably, almost all a total disaster. "Ich liebe dich" is spit and polish fit for the barracks, not the bedroom.

The Casanovan is apt to have verbal communication from his

lady in North American. Which probably can't be helped. But he should still hope to draw something more expressive than rudimentary moans, which he all too readily interprets as ecstasy but may in fact be inspired by a lumpy mattress.

To disesteem CONVERSATION is the mark of the dilettante Lothario. But having an ear for the language of love was by no means the least of the talents that set Casanova above being only a male animal with an exceptionally long rutting season.

Without the verbal pleasure of the prologue, the sex act becomes merely a sketch. Comedic, as often as not.

Aural sex. Casanova knew whereof he spoke. In French. Whose "oui" automatically buds the lips, inviting a kiss.

~ Legs

Casanova was not a legs man. Part of his relative indifference may be attributed to the voluminous frocks and gowns worn by women of his century. He was a great admirer of the shapely foot, on a woman, but from the ankle north was *terra incognita* to his gaze, till it reached the waist. [*See* THIGHS]

His relegating the lower limbs to limbo inspired a celebrated *mot* that Casanova touched off, on the occasion of his guesting in the royal box at the Paris Opera, in company with Madame de Pompadour. The conversation having turned to the comparative study of the dancers' legs, Casanova was heard to remark: "When I am considering the beauty of a woman, *la premiere chose que j'écarte, ce sont les jambes.*" ("The first thing that I set apart is her legs."

The inadvertent pun won him a big laugh, and helped to secure the Venetian's favour with La Pompadour.

In our day of the string bikini it is hard for the Casanovan to ignore a woman's legs, in appraisal of her physical assets. Snug mini skirts are worn even by businesswomen, in their offices and on the public street, and the effect of their crossing their knees, on a man of even normal sexual appetite, can be distracting to the point of his forgetting to breathe.

Combined with stiletto heels, and swathed in dusky shades of hose, our women's legs have become an attention-getting device that would have flipped Giacomo clean out of his gondola.

Yet the incentive to stare must be resisted. Such is the charming perversity of a woman that she deliberately creates an irresistible distraction that she resents having ogled. The split-second timing required of the Casanovan, to avoid appearing gross, would have shocked the man who refined the amorous look to its purest state.

Casanova concentrated that devastating scansion on the lady's upper body. [*See* BREASTS] He could rappel his regard from the most profound cleavage without losing his balance.

However, if the Casanovan finds, after due research, that he is in fact an inveterate legs man, his best recourse is dark glasses. Never mind whether people wonder why you wear them indoors. Or to the Legsaholic Anonymous meeting. And try to raise your sights to a higher horizon.

⸺ Letters

Casanova was a prolific, and eloquent, writer of letters. Including letters to lady loves. In his hand, the pen became the proxy of the penis. The women to whom he addressed his billets-doux saved them as romantic mementos that he recalled, verbatim, for his memoirs.

It is doubtful that a lover can get the same effect with e-mail. Transmission may be speedier, but the print-out lacks the personal touch of handwriting . . . the tear stain . . . the lingering scent of bottled desire . . .

So, it may be well worth a Casanovan wannabe's while to learn to write in longhand, even though it is a struggle to keep the words between the lines. Remember that every woman is an instinctive graphologist. Don't express your ardour in small, cribbed script that will save stationery but lose her interest in a tight spender. A generous, round hand, with modest capitals and open punctuation: that is the effective letter-writing to express your feelings.

Do NOT dot your i's with little hearts. You want to come across as tender, not soppy.

"How do I know what I think till I hear what I say?" That sensible index may be extended to: "How do I know what I feel till I read what I write?" If the Casanovan finds that the effort of writing a letter, to express his undying love, takes more time and consideration of mind than he can spare from watching TSN, then he has a clue to the measurable depth of his affection. The attraction may be only physical. Not a *bad* thing, but not a keeper.

Casanova often supplemented his love letter with a locket, as souvenir of his devotion. In it, his portrait. He obviously saw it as a sound investment, a means to hang around a woman's neck, or better between her breasts, in absentia.

Given legible penmanship and proper postage, the Casanovan's personal letter to his lady will probably stun her, pleasurably, more than any offering she gets on her answering machine.

The pen is still mightier than the sword, and the cell phone.

⇒ Liberation

Casanova was one of the pioneers in the liberation of women. First he liberated them from their clothes, then he freed them of their maidenhood. He treated them as equals, and as often as indicated.

Casanova provided women — hundreds of them — with an irresistible alternative to the patriarchal family. He fathered a lot of children, but never charged the mothers with total care of them. He was long gone before his babies were born. The mothers were free to marry someone more domesticated. Or to become full-time novelists, if they owned a quill.

Living and loving in 18th-century France was the perfect environment for Casanova to enjoy that country's liberation of women. It was a Romanish period of moral decadence (much like today), for nobles and their ladies who got too close to the fun-loving Louis XV. Victorian, they weren't.

These worldly, freewheeling women represented the forerunners of today's career woman. Although restricted to the upper class — common prostitutes being in another category — they enjoyed the beginnings of Eve's freedom to seize the apple without the punishment of having to wear that unflattering fig leaf.

Today the feminist movement has ground to a glacial pace, under scrutiny by women who have detected flaws in egalitarianism. Most obvious of which is the reaction of men — fight or flight — failing to conform to the New Order dictated by the early Greers and Steinems.

It is not the place of the Casanovan, in this controversy, to pass judgment. Pass the wine: that is his contribution to cordial relations. If our women's liberation proves to be a house of cards, so be it. He plays with his own deck. So long as his intentions are honest, i.e. to give and receive pleasure with the liberated woman, with no promise of anything more, he has served with honour in the gender war.

⇝ Lies

Casanova prided himself on being totally honest, with women. With men, it was negotiable. And with the reader of his memoirs, honesty was his creed, as they include a vast amount of unflattering material. Such as, reporting his several bouts of VD, the added-on cost of his dallying with whores.

In his love affairs he respected the principle that, if a man has to cheat to win the game, the victory is hollow. Casanova entered the carnal contest as if the winner would have to take a drug test by God, and be disqualified from the gold medal should his system prove positive for prevarication.

The one to whom he was lying like a sidewalk was his elderly, potty patroness, Mme. d'Urfé, with whom his relations were basically financial, not sexual. He admits that his lies to her "did not even have the merit of probability. A slave of my life of profligacy, I profited by her folly; she was very rich and I did myself much good without doing anybody harm."

When his only objective was sexual pleasure, however, Casanova obeyed a more veracious code. He treated the copulative bed as a space reserved for the truth, as he understood it.

In short, he lied when upright, but was truthful when lying.

The Casanovan will do well to try to meet that ethical standard of levelling with the lady. He must discern the fine line between benign bullshitting — "you are the only woman who ever made me feel like this" — and dirty pool — "my wife turned out to be a lesbian."

Casanova did make allowances: "There are circumstances when a clever man deceives by telling the truth, and such a lie as this must be approved by the most rigorous moralists." (E.g.: "This is the first time I ever made love to a woman, on a trampoline.")

Casanova came on to women as what he was: an internationally recognized rake. The ultimate challenge. He gave none of them reason to believe that he was a candidate for COMMITMENT. For longer than the night shift. When he did speak to them of marriage, he was truly believing this fantasy, so completely that none of his lovers ever reproached him for his having been diverted from the altar by the fickle finger of Fate. That best friend of the philanderer.

In golfing terms: if your sex drive lands you in a bad lie, take the penalty. Don't try to chip out.

⮞ Lingerie

"The pretty nick-nacks I had given her had made her happy; her ardour was redoubled, and the night passed joyously."

Casanova had no hesitation in buying saucy garments for the women he fancied. In fact he took the girl shopping on some occasions, to make sure that she would be putting on something that he would enjoy taking off.

His being at ease in a dress shop will draw the envy of many Casanovans, who tend to panic in the presence of a multitude of wispy panties, teddies, and things consisting of a thong and a price tag.

Because the clerks are always women — usually older women, who can see right through your babbling "I need a present for my wife" (a lie as transparent as the black-lace knickers) — you freeze. The instinctual response is to:

(a) ask "Do you sell men's socks?" or

(b) take flight, by walking straight into a woman's changing room.

Casanova bypassed these blushful imbroglios by the simple expedient of letting his lady do her own shopping, accompanying her, if necessary, to assist in a selection of "nick-nacks." What the gift lost in the element of surprise, the giver gained in preserving a vestige of dignity.

Contrary to feminist propaganda, most women do enjoy receiving totally impractical items from Veronica's Secret. Who can object to receiving evidence that a person relishes the prospect of seeing her virtually naked, in an expensive wisp? Regardless of what her mirror tells her, she has been given a compliment that can be *laundered.*

So, the Casanovan should not be misled into believing that the object of his desire will be more pleased by his giving her the collected works of Germaine Greer. Intellectually, she may feel flattered, but only a very dumb blonde indeed will prefer it to a naughty negligee.

What if the Casanovan is tempted to try the gift lingerie on himself before wrapping it? Another good reason for having your lady do the shopping. Let sleeping togs lie.

∼ Listening

"He who listens obtains."

In just four words, Casanova condenses one of the great truths of a man's success with women.

It is not a hard rule to apply. Most men have two ears, ample for picking up messages spoken across a Starbucks table, or from pillow to pillow. Yet, for too many men, their major infatuation is with the sound of their own voice. They seem to assume that a romantic tête-à-tête is somehow spiced up by their detailed account of the problem they are having with their boss/ ex-wife/ landlord/ income tax assessment/ tennis elbow.

A woman may listen politely to this monologue. She may even take notes, if that makes him feel more expansive, on the couch.

But sooner or later she will be turned off, and be unreceptive to what he tries to say with his hands.

Remember: psychiatrists have no problem getting dates. Because they have learned how to listen. Profitably.

And listening implies hearing. Being able to prick up your ears, like a rabbit, will not satisfy the woman who is saying something she considers important enough to be heard. Verbal intimacy is much more important to women than to men, and the swain who allows his eyes to glaze over, all ears and no savvy, has effectively queered his chances.

Once he has established that he is articulate beyond King Kong, a man should do most of his talking with his eyes. That Casanova had bedroom eyes is beyond dispute. With his gaze, he could lower a woman's eyes and raise her pulse-rate, simultaneously. But he also had the smarts to *listen* when his target spoke, confident that her remarks would be brief enough as to scarcely delay the first kiss.

And once he had sealed her lips with his own, he knew, from vast experience, how to translate her subsequent vocalization — sighs and moans — into the language of love.

❧ Logic

In Casanova's experience, women are rarely addicted to logic. He noted, as a teenager whose first mentor was the priestly Doctor Gozzi, that most of the preacher's congregation were women. To whom faith was more convincing than reason, especially when conveyed by a resonant voice and assured presence.

Doctor Gozzi "condemned thought because it gives birth to doubt." He also detested women, because they represented weakness of the flesh. With such instructions, the intellectually lively

Giacomo could hardly fail to recognize that logic and reason are the key to all the mysteries of life and the universe, except the fair sex.

The greatest marvel of Casanova's career is that he was able to use his intellect to bear on so many follies of religion and government in his time, yet retain his credulity in affairs of the heart.

Here was a man who could trade philosophical volleys with Voltaire, yet be taken in by a common London prostitute. But he never let his being duped by a woman dampen his adoration of the sex. He kept a tight rein on his being reasonable. And surrendered himself, without reserve, to women whose superior instincts he could never hope to match.

Why do so many bright and attractive women become romantically involved with rotters? It defies logic. But it instructs the Casanovan, to pocket his perfectly rational approach to seduction.

Do not be misled by the fact that yon handsome lady has her degree in Engineering and wouldn't be caught dead reading a Harlequin novel. At heart, she responds to the same basic message the dancers and nuns, courtesans and countesses read in the eyes of Mr. Ever Ready.

Save the logic for your analysis of what went wrong — if it will make you feel any better. Which, to be reasonable, is not too likely.

⁓ Looks

"I was not handsome, but I had something better than beauty — a striking expression which almost compelled a kind interest in my favour . . ."

Frederick the Great did not agree. "Do you know that you are a very handsome man?" he told the visiting Venetian, out of the blue, and with no apparent sexual purpose.

Casanova's mirror reported more detail of his compelling facial features: the formidable brow, boudoir eyes, a nose worthy of Caesar's, the sensual mouth, and a chin that promised no resistance to impulse. Too, Chevalier Casanova de Seingalt profited from a tall and athletic build, with reflexes that won him several duels besides those fought in bed.

How important, then, are looks to the candidate Casanovan? If beauty be in the eyes of the beholder, how much must he rely on her having impaired vision?

Regrettably, most young women *are* drawn to the man they describe as "cute." Cuteness is centred in the buns. It extends north to the shoulders and, eventually, the cranial hair. But cuteness is passive. It is no match, even in a crowded room, for the "striking expression" with which Casanova bowled over beauties in much of the known world.

The ultimate power of that expression lay in his regard. Because Casanova was a remarkably intelligent man, with a questing mind that reflected intensity of spirit through the eyes, a woman was ravished before she could even lower her own gaze. The rest of her submission was mere formality — although a nice dinner with wine expedited matters to cinch the victory.

So, it's the look, not the looks, that will engage a kindly interest. Even the short, fat Casanovan may aspire to a tall blonde if his expression conveys something more than brute lust.

Casanova did more than undress a woman with his eyes. His regard created excitement in her mind. Which is why it matters little how expensive are a man's stylish jacket and jeans, if above the neck his expression is cheap.

Love

"God of all nature! — bitter and sweet feeling! Love — charming monster which cannot be fathomed! God who, in the midst of all the thorns with which thou plaguest us, strewest so many roses in our path that, without thee, existence and death would be united and blended together!" — Casanova's passionate invocation of his deity. Illuminated by the candelabra of exclamation points. Clearly, this man was Love's most eloquent apostle.

And his god punishes triflers. Those who believe that they can escape Love's pitiless power, by keeping their relationship with a woman cool and conditional, are doomed to devotion . . .

Despite his perception of the peril, Casanova was captivated again and again. Love's all-day sucker. For this man, love was a divisible power whose parts were as great as the whole.

Casanova knew, as well as any man that ever lived, that the three most dangerous words a guy can say to a girl are "I love you." Strong men have been known to choke, sweat beyond hope of correction by cologne, and sense their nose extending to Pinocchio length, as they force that phrase from their lips. They fear taking the Lord's name — Love — in vain. Even though they believe the words they are uttering to be true, something warns them of horror if they are wrong.

"It is a sort of madness," writes the old Giacomo of love . . . "It is a disease to which man is exposed at all times, no matter at what age, and which cannot be cured . . . Love being a sentiment which cannot be explained!"

A man may be immune to this manic malady, carnal love, yet not be entirely fortunate. Since he is dead.

✒ Machismo

Are women attracted to men who, at first sight or by reputation, come across as dangerous, testosterone-driven, physically menacing adventurers? Of course they are! Silly question.

Nice and mild may get a guy into Heaven, but he'll have to take a number to get a woman's attention.

No, it's not fair. By all rights, Casanova should have been shunned, instinctively, by at least a measurable percentage of the women who set eyes on him. But it appears that only the clinically blind were immune to his fatal attraction, and even they could become affected if they stood close enough to him to feel the vibes from his machismo.

When a woman sized up Casanova, his mien put the stud in study. A muscular six-foot-plus, when he stood up in the theatre or ballroom, left hand poised upon sword hilt, eyes boldly surveying the assembly, no woman present could doubt his reputation of fighting bloody duels, beating up highway brigands as a cardiovascular exercise, and busting out of Europe's premier, escape-proof pokey.

To every woman he presented the ultimate challenge: be the one to tame this gorgeous brute by sheer dedication to her weight-loss program. And she knew that he would defend her honour long after she had lost it in his arms.

So, can the Casanovan hope to achieve the same effect, with hand poised upon hockey stick? Iffy. But at least he can avoid wearing the goalie mask to a party. And try to look as though he expects to score.

Conclusion: the meek may inherit the earth, but till the will is probated, it belongs to the macho.

~ Magic

The chemistry between man and woman is partly alchemy. That is, a woman believes that she can change sexual attraction into commitment, by a means not open to scientific verification. A man thinks that super-heated sex can transform a woman's base motive into a heart of gold.

It's that old black magic.

Casanova used his "supernatural" powers to good effect, with both women and men, solving their problems and fulfilling their dreams with his "pyramids," numerological mumbo-jumbo that worked for him only because the man was phenomenally lucky in anticipating how the cards would fall.

Today's Casanovan may profit from the same credulousness, in the women who, in increasing numbers, are embracing varieties of witchcraft. These Wiccans are the product of feminism that lost its way and ended up in a swamp. What started as a rational movement stuck wildflowers in its hair and tried to exorcise its failures by casting a spell over everything that moves.

It follows — as Casanova well understood — that it is counterproductive to rely entirely on reason and the rational, when seducing such women. One needs only to check out the local casino, to confirm that most of the players cranking the slots or dabbing the bingo card are female, many of them old enough to know that their lucky hat is ineffectual.

As a gender, women are more practical than men, yet are more vulnerable to charms not found on a bracelet. They are a paradox, much to the satisfaction of the Casanovan with wit enough to tolerate eye-of-newt soup in a worthwhile cause.

What is not advisable is to try to impress today's woman by suddenly producing a length of varied-coloured scarf from your mouth. Or inviting her to put handcuffs on you, solely to demonstrate that you can escape them in 30 seconds. Special effects in films and video games have devalued parlour magic as a type of FOREPLAY.

On the other hand, coming across as totally explicable is not something that women find challenging in a man. Down-to-earth is for legumes, gentlemen, not lovers.

～ Marriage

"The grave of love," Casanova called it. More in sorrow than in anger. He showed respect for this last resting place of LOVE, but had no desire to wear the headstone himself.

He never married. Tempted, yes. No man could be in love with so many women, in breath-taking sequence, without at some point risking his straying to the altar, for the ultimate sacrifice of freedom.

For Casanova the gospel regarding marriage was that intoned by Francis Bacon: "He that hath wife and children, hath given hostage to fortune; for they are impediments to great enterprises, either of Virtue of Mischief." Giacomo had no virtuous enterprises to be impeded, but he did dabble in mischief from time to time, usually bed-time.

He also, in the heat of the contest, once actually promised marriage, to the fetching Catarina . . .

". . . We found that we could not wait any longer. Our love for each other was so great that we could not help but let our marriage take place right then."

"'Let God alone receive our mutual pledges,' I said, 'for He knows the purity of our intentions. We will afterwards legalize our tender love with your father's consent, and with the ceremonies of the Church. In the meantime will you be mine, entirely mine?'"

Well, only a real spoilsport would say No. Certainly Catarina leapt at the offer, without realizing that with Giacomo purity of intentions had a short shelf-life.

No doubt Casanova deluded himself as well as his women, regarding the feasibility of his marrying them. And this may be the moral key for the Casanovan:

Promise her anything, so long as you really believe, at the passionate moment, that anything has a chance of happening.

You are under the influence of a mind-altering drug — for "Love is madness," says Casanova. And nobody can be censured for his fantasying marriage while in the throes of that sweet delirium.

Or, failing the excuse of temporary dementia, you can always think of marriage as a minimum security facility.

∾ Masks

As an essential part of the Venetian Wolf's wardrobe, the mask was right up there with the condom. He might dispense with other wear, when scouting the lay of the land, but his attending the carnival or ball with a bare face did not compute.

The mask lent mystery to a woman, too. Of his first assignation with his favourite nun, Marie-Madeleine, Casanova writes:

"My heart was pounding, but seeing it was a man, I avoided him and regretted not having brought my pistols. But the mask, after circling the statue, came to me with outstretched hands. I then recognized my angel in men's clothes . . ."

Thus revved up, Casanova brought even more enthusiasm to the project of removing other items of his angel's garb, including the wings.

The Casanovan has reason to regret the decline of the mask in sexual relations. Today, even bandits don't wear masks. The black balaclava, favoured by robbers of Brink's vans, has never caught on at the prom.

When North American women wear a mask it is mostly to play hockey, or catch softball. A shame. This loss of mystery has made sexual relations a more simply functional exercise.

The mask that gained Romeo admission to the Capulets' ball — where his fatal attraction to Juliet was magnetized — is now a staple at swinger's clubs where husbands and wives are swapped in a sexual orgy that really demeans a romantic disguise.

So, the Casanovan should seize any opportunity to restore the mask — Zorro tolerance? — as a fillip to adventure other than entering a smoke-filled building.

[Note: wearing a mask may require your removing your glasses. If so, do not operate a vehicle.]

⮞ Matchmaking

Today we call it "dumping": the extrication of oneself from a love affair that no longer satisfies the requirements for sheer bliss.

Casanova was a master dumper, in that he could make the termination of a relationship with a woman take on the humanitarian aspect of social work. Thus with the young and relatively innocent Christine:

"Yet I was the slave of sentiment. To abandon the artless, innocent girl was an awful crime of which I could not be guilty. I decided to find her a husband in every way better than me, a husband so good that she would not only forgive me the insult, but also be grateful in the end."

You can't help liking this guy. He goes out of his way to find Christine a handsome young man "of irreproachable conduct" who is happy to wed a beautiful girl who offers not only a seamless reputation but an equally attractive dowry.

"They were married in the church at Preganziol and afterward they both embraced me and told me I was responsible for their happiness."

Beautiful. Brings tears to the eyes of all but the most hardened bachelor.

For the Casanovan, it is a noble ideal: never to brutally dump, but to introduce the erstwhile lover to someone who is a candidate for MARRIAGE. This may require some research, at church picnics and other wholesome social events that you would normally attend only at gun-point.

Naturally, Casanova felt morally obliged to serve as matchmaker only for the youngest and most vulnerable of his conquests. With older, experienced women whose arms and other parts he was leaving, he was much less concerned about finding them a hubby. Especially if they were already married.

With Christine, he was flabbergasted at the ease with which she accepted the transition from his administration to that of her new fiancé. "The reader can imagine . . . my surprise when I saw the young girl calm and perfectly composed! Her calmness dried the tears already gathering in my eyes."

Yes, men *are* more sentimental than women.

Women are cats, happy to define their own territory, without wasting too much emotion on how they got it.

Men are dogs, born rovers, yet relatively soppy about their relationships, and readily fazed by the adaptable feline.

Yet it behooves the Casanovan to act honorably with the woman he is dumping. If he can't fix her up with a spouse, he can at least introduce her to the more stable guys in his martial arts class. Noblesse oblige.

⟋ Mathematics

Casanova was a master of the math of chance. He could have been a great astrophysicist, had he been interested in heavenly bodies other than those he could fondle.

As it was, he was able to dazzle French ministers of finance with his shaping the odds of the national lottery in favour of the state. Which rewarded him with the voucher that funded many of his campaigns against maidenheads.

Casanova also outdid the pharaohs of Egypt in devising pyramid

schemes. Especially for rich women. He never showed much interest in math as an abstract subject. The bottom line he calculated on
wore knickers. Which he hastened to subtract.

Casanova's pioneer work in math, however, has to be his meticulous recording, in the memoirs, of the number of orgasms he reg-
istered in a 12-hour period. [*See* STAMINA]

The Casanovan may well wonder whether a flair for applied
mathematics is somehow connected with scoring with women. Is
math a prerequisite for the Ph.D. (Doctor of Philandering)?

Fortunately, no. The side of the brain that controls deductive
thinking may, however, be connected with the production of male
hormones and some really great sex. This would explain why few
women are attracted to mathematics, as a career. When they have
got a man's number, it is by instinct rather than science.

Both math and womanizing require concentration, if they are to
attain extraordinary levels of achievement. Casanova chose to focus
on sex, and the numbers he put up, while astounding, failed to win
him the esteem garnered by a Pascal or Leibniz.

Our time's greatest mathematician, Albert Einstein, was the
direct opposite of Casanova. He forbade his wife to enter the room
when he was working on the theory of relativity. Casanova would
never have understood that. Being married, that is, not the theory.

Meaning

". . . for women find a meaning for everything."

Almost a throw-away line, yet no message left by Casanova res-
onates more meaningfully for his disciples.

It warns them that a woman scrutinizes every word and action of
her suitor. She will spot at once an iota of bullshit in a profession of
devotion. She can see right through to the fingers crossed behind
the back.

It may help if the Casanovan thinks of himself as a waiter in a
first-class restaurant, who is aspiring to a really big tip.

He is alert to demonstrate to others that this woman with him means more to him than life itself. For instance, by jumping the queue at the theatre box-office . . . walking on the curb side of the sidewalk . . . accepting the invitation to teach him to snowboard . . .

Whether or not a man removes his hat before having sex, it definitely behooves him, meaning-wise, to take off his boots.

What about double meaning *(double entendre)*? I.e. a suggestive word or phrase, too often accompanied by jiggling the eyebrows. Ans: it's a parlour tactic. Sex, for a woman, is a serious matter, at least till the third glass of champagne.

Nowhere in the memoirs do we hear Casanova fooling with his meaning.

Sniggers are for stag parties. Which Casanova never attended, having a 365-day rutting season.

Medicare

Casanova was a pioneer in naturopathic gynecology. Although his cure for frigidity in young women was notable mostly for its high rate of success (99.9%), one of his miracle cures was worthy of Lourdes itself.

Giacomo had just returned to Venice, and was lodging with his friend Dr. Righelini, who was treating the daughter of the widow who owned the building.

"I found myself in the presence of a fine waxen statue. 'She is pretty,'" he comments, "'but the sculptor should give her some colour.'"

Righelini, who has been bleeding this eighteen-year-old beauty, tells Dr. Casanova: the only cure for her would be a good, strong lover. Giacomo recognizes a referral when he hears one. He prescribes bed rest. She goes to bed, and he takes care of the rest.

"All this stunning girl wanted was the Promethean spark," he reports of his own personal shock treatment. "We . . . passed a glorious night, I full of love and the desire of curing her . . ." (The man was all heart.) ". . . and she of tender and ardent passion . . ."

After only three weeks of this nightly regime, "I had the pleasure of seeing her thoroughly cured. I would doubtless have married her, if something most unexpected had not happened . . ."

What happened was that he was thrown into prison. Not for practicing medicine without a license but for other pursuits that offended the Inquisition.

For maladies afflicting older and powerful women, Casanova drew on his metaphysical bag of tricks. With the Duchess of Chartres, for instance, sister-in-law of Louis XV and sufferer of a badly pimpled complexion, his "oracle" prescribed a diet free of liqueurs and ham. De-blotched, the delighted duchess gave him a purse of one hundred louis and "a tortoise-shell box with a very good likeness of herself on it." She couldn't stick with the diet, of course, and broke out in time for her dermatologist to hit the road.

Casanova was also a mole specialist. If a beautiful woman had a fetching mole on her face, he knew — by divination and hands-on experience — where else she would have a mole that needed attention.

"At the entrance of the temple of love," he tells the fair Esther, "you have a mole precisely like that which appears on your chin."

Bingo! With diagnoses like that, the Casanovan can hardly fail to impress, in a class with Johns Hopkins. Pursue your study of female anatomy, sir, but be sure to make notes.

⤳ Ménage-à-trois

Two's company, three's an orgy.

Giacomo tripled his pleasure on several occasions, creating one of the reasons why his memoirs are kept in the part of the public library reserved for serious research . . .

". . . my ardour was increased by Angelique's ecstasy, as for the first time she witnessed the amorous encounter. Lucrezia, dying of her enjoyment, begged me to stop, but as I did not listen to her prayer, she tricked me, and the sweet Angelique made her first sacrifice to the mother of love."

Mistaken identity can be a lot more fun in bed.

In another memorable encounter, with Misses Marie-Madeleine and Catarina: "In a few minutes we were all three in bed and in a state of nature. At first satisfied with enjoying the sight of the barren contest of my two bacchanalians, I was amused by their efforts . . . but soon, excited myself, I threw myself among them, and I made them, one after the other, almost faint away from the excess of love and enjoyment."

One of Casanova's major discoveries, as an explorer of sex, was that it is easier to overcome the diffidence of a woman if another woman is present to set the pace for the mattress marathon.

Nobody wants to be a party-pooper.

The added dimension provided by the threesome (or more-some) is of course that one-on-one intercourse is visually restrictive. The lover is too fully engaged at close quarters to relish all the exciting combinations and permutations of the encounter. Even the bedroom ceiling mirror has its limitations, plus a stiff neck.

Casanova's success with multiple conjugation did, however, depend largely on the youthful, often virginal curiosity of the combo he was part of. The Casanovan should not expect to duplicate the performance, unless he gets really lucky at the church summer camp.

Also, it should always be remembered that Jacques was perhaps the most prodigious sexual athlete ever to come down the pike. And even he was hard put, on occasion, to satisfy the demands of two avid girls in a game with no time-outs.

The realistic Casanovan will dream the impossible dream, but be prepared to pleasure one woman at a go. Especially on bed-springs that are past their prime.

⬥ Mistress

"5 (a) a woman (other than his wife) with whom a married man has a (usu. prolonged) sexual relationship" (*The Concise Oxford Dictionary*)

Casanova never had a mistress, for the good reason that he was never a married man. It is to his credit that, despite his hundreds of sexual relationships, not once did he cheat on his wife. His conscience was clear, in this regard, though he is still rarely cited as an example of moral integrity.

He did of course frequently have sex with the mistresses of other men, including the king of France. He thus avoided the sin of adultery, as well as the punishment of wedlock.

Paris he found to be particularly rich in mistresses, the French having already established *la petite amie* as part of the Enlightenment. As, latterly, the president of the Republic (François Mitterand) has kept a mistress, and had a child by her, without raising a Gallic eyebrow.

It was in the City of Light that Casanova encountered a mistress arrangement that even he found a bit bizarre. The wealthy husband of one of his old girl friends had set his wife up in a separate house, with the understanding that they had supper together every evening. When quizzed about this arrangement, the husband (M. Blondel) explains that he never had a mistress worthy of being a wife, and is now delighted to have a wife worthy of being a mistress.

For the Casanovan, the question of having a mistress is academic, since he will not be getting married in his lifetime. Also, in North America the feminist movement has pretty well rendered the mistress an endangered species of sex partner. Pity.

⊷ Money
"I was successful with both [women] because I was wealthy. Had I been a poor man I should never have known either of them."

Chilling words, for the novice Casanovan who has been hoping to get bags of sex on credit, or on charm alone, or on a desert isle where he has been cast away with a beautiful woman who will take a cheque.

For Casanova, the two most dependable sources of revenue were gambling — a game played on a table — and old barmy Madame d'Urfé, who was game but not rewarding on a table.

His memoirs testify again and again: though money may not buy happiness, it can finance a short-term loan.

So, is it possible to duplicate what this lover extraordinaire accomplished, if the Casanovan is on welfare? Or hag-ridden by paying his taxes? Probably not. Giacomo was fortunate in that the only books of his that the Inquisition audited were naughty books, with pictures. Nor was he under pressure to contribute to a retirement savings plan.

The only bank he dealt with was the faro bank. Where, as the banker, he was assured of hearty earnings so long as he stayed awake longer — i.e. for days — than any of the other players.

This guy had legs — admired by Lady Luck.

The Casanovan's sole advantage: today's liberated woman is often financially independent enough to own her own flat . . . car . . . vibrator. If she really likes him, she may even lend him money, if he signs a few papers.

Ergo, Mme. d'Urfé is reborn! Younger, prettier, more rational. No need for a man to panic into finding a job.

⟁ Mothers

Can be a problem. Over your night of wild sex a mother may raise her frowning face like a clouded moon.

But Casanova nearly always solved the mother problem without having to draw his sword. In a typical episode, he recounts his meeting an actress he knew named Toscani, who is travelling with her "young and pretty daughter." She tells him that her daughter is "a neophyte," and when the duo take exception to his doubting the daughter's virginal integrity, he challenges them to let him test the thesis.

"Thus I was pleasantly engaged for two hours, after which time I was obliged to extinguish in the mother the flames her daughter had kindled in me."

Brilliant strategy. Everyone is satisfied, and presumably a good time was had by all.

The Casanovan who finds himself in the same daughter/mother bind will do well to remember that mamas too have sexual needs. Killing two birds with one stone is not necessarily ecological abuse.

On another occasion, Casanova falls in love (a matter of nano-seconds) with the beautiful young ballet student Agatha. Meeting the girl's mother, "it so happened that I drew the lady into my arms and gave her a kiss. Feeling that she responded and seemed to like it, I went farther, and finally we spent a couple of hours in showing what a high opinion we had of each other." Astonished by her own performance, the smiling matron asks:

"Am I to tell my girl of the way in which you proved to me that you love her?"

Verbal ballet master that he is, Casanova tells her: "if we are not careful to avoid being alone together, what has happened between us will happen often again."

Again, the perfect carrot, for a bunny Mom.

The bottom line: mothers can be managed, Casanovan. *Grandma,* that's the one you've got to watch out for. There are some very horny grannies out there, and they have nothing to lose but their hearing aid.

⌒ Moustache

On the pictorial evidence, Casanova didn't have one. Or a beard. Indeed his entire face appears to have been without shrubbery.

Was the absence of moustache an asset, in his attracting women, or did he succeed as a sexual prodigy despite being naked under the nose?

"It tickles." That is the reaction to be expected from one's date, when the kiss is supplemented by a whisk. Plus a giggle, often. And giggles are contra-indicated, at this stage of love-making.

This surely explains why Casanova, and most men before him and since, have taken literal pains to scrape their face free of fuzz. Daily. And, in his time, without the technological mercy of the electrical shaver or the razor with blades sharp enough to terrify stubble into submission.

True, movie idol Clark Gable is said to have cut a wide swath through Hollywood's womanhood, despite his sporting the lip nap. The exception that proves the rule. More conclusive is that Adolf Hitler — whose record as a lover is spotty to say the least — tried to enhance his charisma with that ridiculous toothbrush. Even Eva hated it.

The moustache did work for Groucho. But not for Neville Chamberlain, who never meant to be funny, adding to the horror of World War II.

Conclusion: behind every moustache lurks a sexually inept villain. ("Ha, ha, me proud beauty!") Better not to look obvious, chaps.

~ Mystery

"Who can she be," I said, speaking to the walls; "this girl who seems to have the most elevated feelings under the veil of the most cynical libertinism?"

Casanova spoke to the walls a lot. The subject matter varied, but his most poignant mural monologues were inspired by women whom he couldn't take in because he couldn't figure them out. Like the queenly Henriette. The woman drove him right up the bedroom wall, by seeming politely indifferent to his tongue hanging out.

Every Casanovan knows the horror of this situation. The obvious he can cope with, whether it be the girl's jumping to wrap her legs around his body, or her coolly leaving the party with the guy she is dating. But the galling question mark? . . .

Having been mystified by the haunting Henriette, Giacomo was then free to concentrate on being totally smitten with this woman smart enough to keep her options open and her legs closed.

In the event, Casanova's affair with Henriette was one of the more enduring, and endearing, of his life. He might easily have married her, had it not been against his principles.

The lesson for the Casanovan: beware the mystery woman who keeps you awake all night without being in your bed. You may be the victim of what Casanova calls "a perfect amorous frenzy." This condition creates not only insomnia but loss of appetite and total indifference to your choice of socks. In extreme cases, your parents or friends may urge you to go to Emergency, because the bags under your eyes have developed handles.

In the worst case of bafflement by woman, the victim will put something in writing. A poem. A song. A letter to the editor of a newspaper, blaming the feminist movement.

Temporary relief only. Better, perhaps, to seek out the easy, open and obliging woman, without mystery of any kind to challenge the Casanovan's slumber. Whether that makes his experience with the sex more complete is a matter of speculation.

⌇ Names

No name, no pack drill.

Casanova expanded on the name game by creating his own impressive sobriquet: Chevalier de Seingalt. "I have taken eight letters," he explained to an enquiring official, "and combined them in such a way as to produce the word Seingalt. It pleased me, and I have adopted it as my surname."

And very effective the name was. Chevalier de Seingalt had doors opened to him — including bedroom doors — that might have been more difficult of entry by plain Jack Newhouse.

For the Casanovan, too, there may be advantages in the assumed name. Using the family name in a romantic adventure can — as Romeo found out — cause problems. Some of them fatal. So, unless he anticipates taking the lady home to meet Mom and Dad, there is no reason why the Casanovan should not adopt a surname that falls well on the feminine ear.

A stellar example: one of the early premiers of British Columbia, born William Smith, took the name Amor de Cosmos (Love of the Universe) and never looked back. Would simple Bill Smith have cut as fine a figure?

And though Archie Leach might still have become one of films' most romantic idols, as Cary Grant he had a better shot.

The tradition that a man should bear his father's surname has been eroded by custom. Fathers come and go, these days, often replaced by the dads of new family relationships. As Casanova pointed out to the official: "Your name . . . cannot be more true than mine, for it is possible that you are not the son of the gentleman you consider your father."

Don't try that one on a Customs officer, but in other circumstances the Casanovan should feel free to be creative if the woman he is dating asks him his name. Although our popular music has established "Baby" as the generic name for both genders on the make, some women want a name they recognize on their voice-mail.

Suggestion: "Chevalier de Seingalt." (Chances are, the lady will not recognize the name as Casanova.) "But you can call me 'Chevy.'"

All's fair in love and war — if indeed one can distinguish between those two perilous arenas.

➪ No!

The most dreaded word in the libertine's lexicon. The more so for often being (a) unspoken, or (b) easily misheard as "maybe," or (c) yelled loud enough to shatter a windshield.

Hard to believe though it is, Casanova did once have a violent collision with the negative, erected by a woman he had wangled into the sheets. It makes tragic reading. No man who has been thwarted at the height of his ardour can read them without dabbing his eyes . . .

"It was a dreadful night. I spoke to this monster of a woman in every manner and tone — with gentleness, with argument, rage, remonstrance, prayers, tears and abuse, but she resisted me for three hours without abandoning her painful position, in spite of the torments I made her endure." Oh, the agony! "I felt tempted to strangle her; and then I knew it was time for me to go."

Well, Casanova did know when to take a hint. Which is to his credit, though when he went home, he couldn't sleep, and developed a fever, and was deathly ill for days.

If this could happen to our hero, it behooves every Casanovan to recognize that when a woman assumes the fetal position, as if to defend against a plane crash or earthquake, and remains in that frozen attitude for hours at a time, she really is disinclined to receive him.

A blow to the male ego, yes. A kick in the groin as painful as anything delivered by Jackie Chan. But the Casanovan will do himself a favour by discarding any self-assessment he may have made as being irresistible to the unfair sex. Chances are that, unlike Alexander the Great, he will not be weeping because there are no new women to conquer.

"No!" (or "Non" or "Nein" or "Nyet" etc.) may be the last word he misinterprets before hearing that the speaker has charged him with sexual assault. Yes, rape. Doubly hurtful when all he got was a throbbing headache.

So, one must respect "No!" unless a moan invites clarification. Yet one should not be *too* responsive to a No, as this may affront the lady as an insult to her charm. Having ABS braking on your sex drive does not impress the woman looking for a Grand Prix winner.

Such was his expertise in FOREPLAY that Casanova had rare occasion to have to deal with ugly Nos. And the fact that he chronicled his come-uppance as faithfully as he did his world-record for yesses, gives us reason to pay homage to his objectivity. No?

Nomadism

Military historian John Keegan, writing of the life of the North American Indian, observes that the nomad "enjoys the greatest of all human endowments, personal freedom and detachment from material burdens. Nomadism, anthropologists have concluded, is the happiest of all human ways of life."

Casanova was the happy nomad personified. He didn't have a stationary moment in his life, other than his months in prison, where travel was necessarily limited, and in his old age, when he lost it in the legs.

For all the rest of his yeasty years he was the soul mate of the plains Indian of America. Instead of following the great herds of buffalo, Casanova toured the courts of Europe, picking off game with feckless ease.

Especially the fair game.

Giacomo extended the roving eye to all parts of his body. He would envy his disciples' benefits of modern transportation, as the automobile and airplane have made nomadism much more comfortable than in the days of horse and carriage. There is no excuse for the Casanovan to be stuck in one town, with all the temptations that immobility presents, including the most deadly: *settling down.*

Dregs settle down. All that remains of the wine of sex life.

Casanova showed that a woman is much more susceptible to seduction by a travelling man than by a person who lives in her neighborhood. Her reputation is less at risk, when her lover is living out of a suitcase. Thus in the classic motion picture "Brief Encounter," we recall, one of the main romantic characters is the train.

By rail, air or cruise ship, the Casanovan will meet countless women hungry for romantic adventures. The same women, on their home turf, will be looking for a mate to share the responsibilities of home and hearth — and there goes Sitting Bull, into the freezer.

True, Casanova could afford to travel fecklessly from boudoir to boudoir because he was sponsored financially by a wacky old woman. But today we have the National Hockey League, the pro golf circuit, the trucking industry and other surrogates for Madame d'Urfé.

The blithe spirit of the Sioux Indian can still be attained, and with better room service than a teepee.

❧ Novels

"Most likely the reading of a certain class of novels causes the ruin of a great many girls, but I am of opinion that from good romances they acquire graceful manners and a knowledge of society."

Casanova was endorsing the "good" novels of his time. Would he have found the same source of "graceful manners" in today's Chick

Lit? Perhaps not. Most men are ignorant of what goes on in these enormously popular bodice rippers, and that may be a mistake. It could well serve the Casanovan to research the latest Harlequin novels, so long as he doesn't do it on the bus. Wearing an old raincoat.

Breaking the enemy's code is a covert operation.

What the Casanovan will learn form the women's novel is that romance is still an essential part of their enjoyment of sex. This principle was well understood by our grand master, who instinctively blandished his objectives with lavish dinners, grand social occasions, and pricey gifts, even going to the trouble of buying them pretty clothes other than the inevitable black-lace lingerie that is the wrong size.

This doesn't mean that the Casanovan should study the 18th-century works of Mme. de Scudéry, or Samuel Richardson's *Pamela.* Time has marched, or rather sashayed, on, in feminist novels. They are considerably more sexually explicit, while satisfying fantasies that may be too extravagant for the guy who is working on a tight schedule.

But Casanova himself never begrudged the time to acquaint himself with the secret desires of the women as disclosed by their novels. Remember: Harlequin was Casanova's favourite guise, when setting forth to cruise the do of the evening. Putting all his cards on the table was something he reserved for his other games of chance. For women, he presented the figure of mystery that their romances today still project as the Real Deal.

No need to buy the wretched things. Try your local public library. Just wear dark glasses.

☙ Novelty

"Novelty is the master of the soul." (Casanova here assumes the existence of the soul, even in the most libertine of bodies.) "We know that what we do not see is very nearly the same as what we have seen, but we are curious, we like to be quite sure, and to attain our end we give ourselves as much trouble as if we were certain of finding some prize beyond compare."

He is talking about women. Looking back with the wisdom of the sexually impotent, he sees that he has devoted much of his considerable energy to exploring territory that was already well mapped: *La Femme*. This he did with no hope of claiming a place in history beside Magellan or Galileo, by discerning a woman with more than two charming breasts, or whose pubic hair concealed a rare treasure worthy of Hindu mythology.

Today, the Casanovan may be tempted to dally with a dominatrix — a sexual aberration that Giacomo apparently had no occasion to investigate. But whether she wears leather or lace, the physiognomy of woman is basically standard. In the dark — as the cruel adage goes — all women look alike. Knowing this, every woman strives to look as different, in the light, as she can, from every other woman, within the bounds of fashion. She willingly feeds the male's hunger for novelty, expecting that the unique features of her mind will win his constancy. Or at least a free beer.

And this can actually happen. Yes, even to a devout Casanovan.

As our retired roué notes, indefatigable curiosity cost him as much trouble and anxiety as if he were sweating in the jungle in search of a new species of wild-cat — with no hope of ever finding one.

In the interest of self-preservation, therefore, the Casanovan will heed the belated conclusion drawn by our mentor, by limiting his hunt for novelty in women, and will expend more of his physical/mental resources on attaining, say, a novel variety of putter. Or power-tool.

In short, novelty doesn't age well. Neither, as it happened, did the Chevalier de Seingalt. Whom the gods love die young — just to complete their novel experiences.

∾ Nudity

Venturing into a public bath in Berne, Casanova is greeted by a swarm of young women bidding to attend him in his ablutions. He selects one, who undresses him, gets naked herself, and in the bath gives him a vigorous scrub-down which, on paper, should have had the opposite effect to a cold shower.

It didn't. "But why did I remain cold to her charms?" he asks rhetorically. His answer: "Probably because she was too natural, too devoid of those assumed graces and coquettish airs that women use with so much art to seduce men."

The girl refuses his tip, offended because he failed to find her an arousing experience.

Casanova's was one of the earlier experiments to establish that nudity can be a sex depressant. It may turn men off, and women find it hilarious. If Adam and Eve had not sinned in the Garden, and thus been made aware of their nakedness, and therefore obliged to wear the fig-leaf, mankind might never have generated. Cancelled because of lack of interest.

On another watery occasion, Casanova takes his date to one of Moscow's public baths, there to dunk with thirty or forty women and men, "quite naked, but as no one looks at anyone else, he fancies he is not seen by anybody but himself."

Similarly a German spa proves to be an anaphrodisiac to this Italian endowed with a spirited imagination. Again and again, in his romantic encounters, what enthralls Giacomo is a "glimpse" of some part of a beauty's anatomy that wasn't supposed to be visible.

The inference we may draw: women may have done themselves a disservice, as sex objects, when they divested their body of crinolines. Except for the *Sports Illustrated* swimsuit models, few women profit from being seen nude in broad daylight. And Casanovans are suckers for MYSTERY. When they go to the striptease bar, it's the tease that provides the ignition.

The naked bottom line: do not seek romance in a nudist camp. Instead, visit those Asian lands where women still wear the sari, the chador, the cheongsam. You will learn why those lands are so heavily overpopulated, and the men look very relaxed.

🖎 Occupation

Casanova proved that having a steady job is not a plus factor in philandering. On the contrary, occupational stability encourages women to consider a man as a potential *breadwinner*. Winning bread is contra-indicated for the Casanovan, much as he may enjoy a warm, crusty loaf. He may also find himself sinking roots, which can fatally impede the mobility so essential to the career womanizer.

Casanova never went to the office. The office may be defined as a man-trap with lousy coffee. Its cubicles and warrens are mined, with either a charge of sexually harassing a fellow employee, or COMMITMENT to Ms. Millstone in Accounting. Going to the office (the Oval Office) caused disaster for President Bill Clinton, who might have been remembered as one of the great American presidents, had he worked from home.

Casanova, however, had his priorities straight. He avoided work anywhere. His resumé would show that his first job, as an abbé, into which he was led while still too young to understand the threat to dissipation, he escaped quite unscathed by a work ethic. From then on, he became a professional friend of the rich and powerful (both sexes), as well as a poet, playwright, alchemist, necromancer, military officer (self-appointed), mathematician and the ultimate gypsy.

He never had to concern himself with public relations, because his private relations gave him all the reputation he needed to be welcomed into high society, whose credo was *"le seul péché, c'est d'ennuyer."* ("The only sin is to be boring.")

Casanova was a travelling salesman who sold himself — to the high, the mighty, and the yummy.

But what a product he did offer! Such an array of talents would be called Promethean, had he stolen fire as well as other means of keeping warm in bed.

Gifted indeed will be the Casanovan who can accomplish even a fraction of the master's work-free feats. We are all so busy providing for our retirement that we forget to plunder the present.

The nerve has been killed by political correctness. Yet for the man who dares to live with one hand on the sword and the other on a perky breast, ours is still an inviting environment. The Internet beckons the freelance spirit, though it will never compete with the open range of Jacques Casanova, till the modem mouse can return a loving caress.

✍ Old Age

". . . What embitters my old age is that, having a heart as warm as ever, I have no longer the strength necessary to secure a single day as blissful as those which I owed to this charming girl."

The wolf in winter. For the Casanovan, too, there comes a time when, though he turns for help from the saviour (Viagra), he cannot muster the sexual vigour of his salad days. Like the sun and death, this prospect is one that no young man can contemplate.

Women wear better. For men, especially, growing old is the pits. Of despair. Even the happily married codger has problems with his plumbing that cause his eyes to water as he thumbs through the copy of *Playboy* magazine in the barber shop, there where the damnable distorting mirrors aggravate his image of balding decrepitude.

What to do? How can the Casanovan prepare for this period of his life — and now he could live to a hundred — when any interest he evinces in the opposite sex earns him the title "silly old goat"?

For Jacques the answer — by no means as "blissful" as his romantic adventures — was writing. His memoirs, his letters to old friends (including girl friends), these helped to assuage the ravages of old age.

When he could no longer get it up, he put it down. On paper. That submissive victim of so much vicarious sex.

The Casanovan who derives no satisfaction from writing should prepare an alternative reason for staying alive after sixty-five. Men who work with their hands, on material other than fair flesh, have the advantage over professionals, who in their desperation may marry much younger women who esteem them for their yacht. Mr. Hugh Hefner, publisher of *Playboy,* is the role model for this class of greying Casanovan, but to get started in the girlie mag business requires resources beyond those photos one took of Mabel at the beach last summer.

The Internet's chat lines, of course, can provide the antique Casanovan with electronic intercourse with younger women working with older computers. But visual web sites spell doom for all but the old man in the iron mask croaking endearments through the grille.

The sad truth is that, for the Casanovan even more than for other men, "the golden years" are solid lead, painted yellow by vendors of insurance policies.

So, gather ye rosebuds while ye may, laddie, as the future is rife with thorns.

⌇ Older Women

"She always appeared young, even in the eyes of the best judges of faded, bygone female beauty . . ."

Casanova here is reporting on the remarkable French dancer Binetti, whose latest lover she killed "by excess of amorous enjoyment," at the age of sixty-three.

"Men . . . are right in not racking their brain for the sake of being convinced that they are the dupes of external appearance." Casanova himself was free of prejudice against older women, as lovers, though he never risked suicide by trying to satisfy a randy sexagenarian. Purely a one-time investment deposit: that was his humping Madame d'Urfé, the old moneybag who challenged his capacity for arousal so severely that he needed a hooker in the adjoining room, to prime the pump.

In the absence of a retirement savings plan as we know it, Casanova was providing for his financial future.

The Casanovan has a wider, and younger, selection of mature, wealthy ladies. Females are now business executives, owners of their own prosperous commercial enterprises. Typically, such an older woman now has the job she wanted, and owns the Land Rover SUV she wanted, and is now in the market for a boy toy, a stud to take to Maui for a romantic lei.

At least, that is how it should work in theory. Why wouldn't a man welcome sex with a woman of sufficiently advanced years to eliminate the hazard of child support, or the paternity suit, and that bugaboo of so many eagerly anticipated weekends: the Period?

The Casanovan who has misgivings about being part of abortion on demand should, one would think, confine his foraging for sex to annual shareholders' meetings . . . community centre bowling . . . garden clubs. And forget his glasses.

But he doesn't. The promise of more stimulating conversation with the older woman, the easy sharing of the restaurant bill, the (possibly) sexual expertise that diversifies positions beyond the prostrate and frozen missionary — these fail to divert most Casanovans from the pursuit of the giggly young thing.

The Life Force makes fools of us all. All one can do, as a Casanovan, is to make the reproductive imperative as mutually enjoyable as possible. She's a bitch, that Mother Nature.

❧ Onanism

"Is onanism a crime amongst you?" Casanova asks a Turk Muslim philosopher.

"Yes, even greater than lustful and illegitimate copulation."

Casanova begs to differ: "A man in good health, if he cannot have a woman, must necessarily have recourse to onanism, whenever imperious nature demands it, and the man who, from fear of polluting his soul, would abstain from it, would only draw upon himself a mortal disease."

The Turk counters with the argument — still heard today — that "young people shorten their lives through self-abuse." Or at least soon need coke-bottle eyeglasses.

Casanova's riposte: "If girls are not interfered with in the matter of self-abuse, I do not see why boys should be."

The Turk: "What they lose does not come from the same source whence flows the germinal liquid in men."

Read: thou shalt not spill thy seed upon the ground. Or — if thou should hope to escape damnation on a technicality — in the toilet.

Casanova called it "manustupration." The last resort of the schoolboy. No one knows how much onanism — nervously derided as "wanking" — is practiced by either gender today. Stats Can has no figures, and may not even return your call.

But the popularity of porno videos and strip bars would indicate that many men are settling for second best, by way of answering one of Mother Nature's less spiritual calls.

On the positive side, Jacques' defence of (no relation) jacking off jibes with the counsel of most family physicians: that mighty generative motor in your jockey shorts should have the oil changed fairly regularly, or nasty conditions can total the whole vehicle. Ideally, you won't offend Allah or Jehovah, but you can't please everybody.

The Casanovan who feels guilty about having a one-man party should console himself with the thought that, if onanism were more respected, we would all be paying less taxes for social services to abortion clinics, unwed teenage moms, and other hidden costs of "making out" as a rite of passage.

A reliable vibrator costs less than the dinner for two at an expensive restaurant (including tip), and the relatively minor expenditure of time and emotional energy improves one's chances of making the school soccer team.

Casanovonanism. For quick relief only, never a substitute for the romance that includes a member of the opposite sex.

～ Opportunity

". . . for I was persuaded that a lover is lost if he does not catch fortune by the forelock."

Casanova had a quick hand to the lady's forelock, if not other fortuitous tufts. He well understood that, with a desirable woman, he who hesitates is lost, or at least mislaid.

It seems cruel, but the shy, reticent applicant for a woman's favour loses out to the bold, self-assured bounder. Being overly cocky can, of course, conduce to an impromptu appointment with an orthodontist. Indeed, it is a very fine line, indiscernible to many of us, between the gross opportunist and the faint heart that ne'er won fair lady.

The most common indicator of opportunity is flirting. Women do flirt, though often so subtly that a man mistakes the come-hither smile for gas. Or, worse, what he sees as a flirtatious wink may be an optic tic. So that his responding wink is in very poor taste, if not fatal.

On balance, however, it is better to err on the side of assumption of opportunity, so long as your personal insurance is paid up. A woman will forgive your responding to an invitation that isn't there, more readily than to your ignoring one that is.

Casanova well understood that a young woman, in company, is always "on." She may be happily married and accompanied by her husband, yet she is constantly aware of the effect she is having on any and all males within eyeshot. The teenage prom, or rave, is the proving ground for this never-ending mating ritual, in which the male is expected to be overt, the female more selective.

Thus, the novice Casanovan who is subject to having other matters on his mind — such as swimming, when at the beach, or listening to the lecture, when in the classroom — may fumble fortune's forelock.

Not so, Jacques. When Opportunity knocked, he already had his hand on the door-knob, ready to admit a new romance. And she does, remember, only knock once.

ᷓ Oysters

To soften up a woman's defensive position, the shelling of the oyster has long been a favourite ordinance. Second only to the alcoholic punch. Both of which, in combination, Casanova employed as a superlative tactician.

As when he took on the two nuns, Armeline and Emilie, with his dinner party game . . .

"We ate fifty oysters, and drank two bottles of sparkling champagne . . . I placed the shell on the edge of her lips, and after a good deal of laughing she sucked in the oyster, which she held between her lips. I instantly recovered it by placing my lips on hers . . ."

(Obviously a great ice-breaker, for any private party: the roistering oyster.)

"This gave me the opportunity of teaching them the game of tongues, which I shall not explain because it is well known to all true lovers . . . It so chanced that a fine oyster slipped from its shell as I was placing it between Emilie's lips. It fell on to her breast, and she would have reclaimed it with her fingers; but I claimed the right of regaining it myself, and she had to unlace her bodice to let me do so . . ."

A versatile mollusc, the oyster. There's no telling where it will slither to, between friends.

Before the Casanovan rushes out to buy a bushel of oysters, he should understand certain rules of the oyster-exchange game, which can be disastrous for the amateur:

– Do not try this at home. Oyster supping, sipping and sucking can make a mess of your dining area, with slippery footing and shells in your sofa. Rent a hall. Or at least a hotel room. Best of all, have your oyster party at the beach. Where even the oysters will feel more at home.

– Forget the myth that oysters contain a natural aphrodisiac. This shellfish has no more credentials than the common clam. It just looks, feels and smells sexy. Otherwise it is as innocuous as granola.

– Swallowed raw, the oyster can ruin any party if affected by red tide, or if the chef opened the shell with a rusty shoehorn. A trip to Emergency is no post-prandial picnic.

– Should your guest find a pearl in her oyster, let her keep it. Don't spoil the mood. If she finds a whole string of pearls, start dating your fishmonger.

[Note: the prairie oyster (a raw egg yolk) is not as romantically effective with women beyond the plains.]

⤳ Paris

It's a truism: every man has two home towns: his own, and Paris.

The same may be true for every woman, but it is a less documented fact of demographics.

"Paris the Only, Paris the Universal," exults Casanova the Amatorian, describing his first visit to the city on the sinuous Seine. Fortune's playground. "The only town where the blind goddess freely dispenses her favours."

He meets there a fellow Italian refugee from honest work, Count Tiretta of Trevino, whom Casanova introduces to Madame de Lambertini, a wealthy widow with whom Tiretta spends the night and receives the title (bestowed by his accommodating hostess) of "Count Sixtimes." An award earned by her guest's "erotic achievements."

When queried about the origin of the title, Casanova explains: "My friend in a single night did what a husband often takes six weeks to do."

Such statistics were based on Casanova's own research into the remarkable enhancing effect of Paris on the libido. He returned to the city again and again, made it his veritable base of operations against the most sexually savvy women in Europe.

Perhaps the prairies of North America can boast that never is heard a discouraging word, but Paris has been even more positive — home of the cancan, in fact.

So, what is it about Paris that can turn a visitor into a conjunctive Superman, without his having to waste time changing in a phone booth?

The mystique has for centuries drawn visitors (mostly male) from other countries such as Britain, where sex, when it occurs at all, is something of an anomaly. Paris has been the creative mecca of North American novelists, from Miller to Mailer, eager to shake off the inhibitions of Main Street, U.S.A. This regardless of the price of a cup of coffee in a Boulevard Montparnasse bistro.

Why is "gay paree" such a metropolitan aphrodisiac?

Well, the city is well-rounded. Topographically, Paris *rues* are a bosomy series of curves, girdled with the green ribbon of the Seine. Seen from the air, she is "La Courtesane" rendered large. Hilly San Francisco and Vancouver, British Columbia, do their best to compete with Parisian pulchritude, but the grid system discourages the roving eye.

A guy visiting from, say, Toronto, Ontario (on that straight-laced lake) can start to feel horny just standing on the Pont Neuf and watching the Seine flow curvaceously to wherever it wants to go.

Inevitably, the tallest structure in Paris has been a naked erection. The eyeful Tower. No one who beholds it can remain unmoved, usually towards the Folies Bergère.

Every devout Casanovan must make the pilgrimage to Paris, to complete his sexual education. Don't wait till you are on your honeymoon. See Naples and die. See Paris and live!

◀ Passions

"When it is a question of an affair of the heart, of the passions, or of pleasure, a woman's fancy moves much faster than a man's."

This acceleration — of a woman's passion, that is — can startle the Casanovan who is not prepared for it. As in the lift-off of the space shuttle, he may experience G-force that pins him to his car's bucket-seat/ the park bench/ the boat deck. His cheeks compress, his eyes bug, and he may lose consciousness if he forgets to breathe.

A man's passion, in contrast, is more likely to be a smooth if not gradual continuum, a sort of automatic transmission of emotion. Some men do gear up manually, seeing themselves as a sports model lover, but most are conscious of the fine line between the acceptable progress of passion and sexual assault that is a criminal offence.

Women have no such braking. As Casanova attests from his encyclopedic knowledge of the sex, their fancy can zoom from zero to flat out in a matter of seconds.

This is why the Casanovan must beware of starting something that he doesn't expect to leave the garage. [*See* HUMBUG] Today's woman is even faster to put the pedal to the metal of her lust. Her time is valuable, more so than in Casanova's society. Although she may not become sexually aroused as quickly as her partner, during what he fondly admires as his artful foreplay, he can suddenly find himself lapped, and forced to make a pit-stop because he has blown a tire.

Woman's passions, unfortunately, do not come with an air-bag.

Pedophilia

If she's big enough, she's old enough.

This criterion for sexual intercourse was sedulously observed by Casanova, during his extended romp through *Le Pays de l'Amour*. He does not hesitate, in his memoirs, to include a girl's tender age, along with the other specs for his being enthralled. The fourteen-year-old was quite eligible. (He was occasionally tempted by a pre-teen, but the lisp turned him off.)

The early harvesting of maidenhead — Casanova's forte — was to be expected in a period when the average lifespan was 35 years. Compared to our time, all the stages of life were accelerated, and Giacomo set the pace for overtaking the virgin. Had he known that he would live into his seventies — the equivalent of hitting a hundred today — he might have slowed to savour more of the mature woman. But it is hard to imagine why.

The Casanovan has no such options. Sex with a minor is a serious crime in western society, and the pedophile is not welcome in any neighborhood where the children are allowed out of the house. A game not worth the scandal.

What if the Casanovan is himself a teenager who finds himself being fondled by an older woman? This dilemma is more prevalent than in earlier days, before the school-teacher had her own apartment. Or before the choir leader drove the boy soprano home and made him a basso before they got there.

Is the kid's life ruined by this experience? His lawyer may nod Yes, but much depends on how the predatory female is built, and how readily she lets him access her Palm Pilot, as well.

Most youthful Casanovans will be sensible to accept that they have been gravely despoiled, stop giggling and get on with their lives. However, trauma therapy is available, often offered by a good-looking social worker who believes in the curative power of hugging.

Once he reaches the age of twenty-one, though, the Casanovan should not expect to receive financial compensation for being sexually abused by an older woman. Jacques himself would be the first to confirm that falling victim to a voracious manizer helps to build character. Among other benefits.

⤳ Perversion

"'What! You do not love him, and yet you make use of him in the way you do.'"

"'Yes, just as I might make use of a mechanical instrument.'"

"In this woman I saw an example of the depths of degradation to which human nature may be brought."

Yes, Casanova was shocked. He had just watched this woman (Nina) having sex with her drunken consort, a spectacle that so disgusted him that he had to refuse her invitation to make her evening more interesting. She protests:

"I only use him to satisfy my desires, and because I am certain that he does no love me."

"Words," comments the astonished Giacomo, "that I had never heard a woman use before." Words that had the effect on him of a cold shower.

To this man who worshipped women, it was blasphemy. From a whore he might expect this perversion of the loving relationship. But this was a "respectable" lady. Having sex with a pickled partner as a mere utility.

"I had known women of similar character, but never one as dangerous as she."

This perverse breed of broad is by no means an endangered species. If anything, sex can be even more inconsequential for today's liberated women than for the nasty Nina.

While the Casanovan may never encounter a woman who uses him as a joyless sex aid, he should always be alert to seduction by a harpy.

He should beware any circumstance or social event where a very attractive woman encourages her escort to get drunk, while she comes on to the Casanovan. As the Great One warns: she may be uncommonly dangerous. The woman who abuses sex as mere physical exercise may challenge the romantic Casanovan to try and light a fire amid cold ashes. And get burned.

Casanova did eventually overcome his revulsion at the nubile Nina — by beating her at cards. When you have taken a woman's money, and she still wants you for a lover, you may be sure that the experience cannot be a total loss.

⤨ Pity

"When we can feel pity, we love no longer . . ."

Casanova took care not to give any woman cause to pity him. When thwarted — which did happen with a few ladies having strong principles or weak impulses — his response was to vigorously accuse the resister of being impaired by unnatural inhibitions.

Never did he whine, pout, threaten suicide or otherwise try to induce pity. Which he saw to be the killer of amatory desire.

The man who sees pity shining in the eyes of the woman he desires is, for all practical purposes, dead. The Dear John letter is in the mail. It will express sorrow that the relationship has passed on, and may bear insufficient postage.

Men's support groups depend heavily on the membership of guys who assumed that the woman they craved would take pity on them. These losers may even have learned how to weep openly, in her presence, in the mistaken belief that the fire of passion will burn stronger if watered by tears.

To be pitied by a woman *before* sex therefore is a downer that the Casanovan must avoid at all costs. It can cause erectile dysfunction for as long as a week. And the only defence against it — as Casanova demonstrated to perfection — is a sturdy ego. One that operates on the basic premise that a woman's REJECTION of him is proof that:

 (a) her eyesight is badly compromised, or

 (b) she is a latent lesbian, or

 (c) her answering machine is deceased.

Whether or not the Casanovan's woman is more to be pitied than censured, he should strive to ensure that he doesn't invite her commiseration. That is why it is so important to have other legitimate accomplishments, as did Jacques, to insulate his self-esteem against pity.

Not inclined to fighting duels to the death? Well, try league bowling.

∾ Playwriting

Casanova tossed off stage plays as casually as other men write a laundry list. He appears to have been attracted to the stage early on, not as a forum for ideas but as the best place to meet actresses. Ladies of the theatre, then as now, were not noted for their moral rectitude. Also, they were apt to be pretty. The perfect environment for the creative lecher.

And Jacques was a fast playwriter. "I spent several days," he reports, "translating Voltaire's *L'Ecossais* into Italian for the actors at Genoa to play." What he wrought in less than a week earned him a bad review from the great French philosopher, but of more immediate concern was the play's opening night — without a prompter. Casanova volunteers to fill in:

"I will occupy the box myself," he tells one of the actresses, but I shall see your drawers."

"You'll have some difficulty in doing that," remarks another actor. "She doesn't wear any."

"So much the better."

As an added perk, the play sold out for the entire run, and got good notices everywhere but at Ferney.

For the Casanovan, the incentive to participate in theatre, whether as playwright, prompter or stagehand, amateur or pro, on Broadway or Noway, is that:

Actresses think of clothes as a costume. Something to be readily taken off, if the act requires it.

Also, all good actors are essentially characterless, their art depending on their ability to assume another identity. With Casanova's enormous talent for making a woman feel like a queen, the actress was most readily coronated on the cot.

Conclusion: of all genres of creative writing, the stage play is the most productive, socially. You may have to build your own theatre to get your play produced, but nobody ever said that great sex comes cheaply.

[Note: whatever he does, the would-be Casanovan should not write novels. The novelist's is the loneliest literary activity on earth. The only drawers he gets to see are in his desk.]

➤ Pleasure

That Casanova dedicated his entire life to pleasure — especially sexual pleasure — is obvious to the reader of his memoirs. One can only be overwhelmed with admiration for his resolve to avoid any activity, such as a steady job, that was not focussed on pleasure. Truly, this was an imperative calling. Nay, a mission.

What is not understood so well is how much pleasure he gave to others. Witty and gracious, he was the life of any party. The pleasure he provided in company won him the favour of kings and queens, as well as young ladies whose treasures were not kept in palace halls.

But of course the latter were his greatest source of *pleasure*. He defines the technique of titillation:

"If the seducer is clever the young innocent will soon have gone too far to be able to draw back. Before she has time to think, pleasure attracts her, curiosity draws her a little farther and opportunity does the rest."

Casanova — an amateur philosopher at best — does not appear to have pondered the question of whether sexual pleasure is the way Mother Nature — ever fixated on reproducing the species — tricks us into performing an act that we might otherwise pass up in favour of a lively game of Scrabble. Or just a snooze on the sofa.

Historian Michel Foucault records the tortured philosophical debate on this subject, which has teased thinkers since the ancient Greeks started asking questions that can ruin your evening.

For instance: Galen et al identified aphrodisia — i.e. sensory turn-ons — as the guilty party in our finding sex more fun than, say, taking out the garbage.

"The approach he recommends is clearly Stoic" writes Foucault (in *The History of Sexuality,* vol. 3 "The Care of the Self"): "it is a matter of considering pleasure as nothing more than the accompaniment of the act; it must never be taken as a reason to accomplish the act."

But is it the Stoic that delivers babies? (Yes, it had to be asked.)

Galen also cites the exemplary sexual behaviour of spawning fish, which discharge their sperm without any visible sign of having a jolly good time. No wonder the Greeks got slogged by the Romans.

No Stoic he, Casanova was motivated by the prospect of pleasure every time he made love to a woman (Mme. d'Urfé excepted). He never stopped in mid-smooching to ask himself: "Am I doing this only because I am programmed to perpetuate my species regardless of whether I would sooner be banging a drum?"

In this matter of sexual pleasure, not Greeks but geeks are today's guys — lamentably the product of North American culture — who regard as perversion anything that makes a woman feel good. It is not uncommon for them to make love with their eyes shut, lest they see something that might shock them.

Yet any man who has (inadvertently of course) glimpsed an explicit video knows that it is the expressed ecstasy of the woman that turns him on, not the grunting grimaces of the male.

In bed, too, 'tis more blessed to give than to receive . . . pleasure. So long as he observes this simple credo, the Casanovan — regardless of how many women he has seduced — can live comfortably with his conscience.

~ Poems

From start to finish of his long career as a philogynist, Casanova wrote ardent poems to the women he fancied, having discovered, early on, that as an entrée to a woman's heart, verse is second only to body language. Especially when combined with a really fine wine.

Don't boggle, Casanovan. Although many, if not most, young men today consider writing poetry to be sissy stuff, a means of expression best left to mentally tortured females with bird's-nest hair and a sour attitude, the fact remains that a traditional love poem — written by hand on unlined paper — is indisputable proof of the suitor's willingness to go to the trouble and expense of buying a rhyming dictionary.

Let us not be deceived by the decline of romantic expression. Talking dirty on the Internet chat-line is no substitute for a sensitive sonnet, or even a quivering quatrain.

Actually, rhyme is not a requisite — as it was in Casanova's day —

for an effective poem. Anything tiered in short lines — (don't skimp on paper) — now qualifies as verse. The main purpose is to delight the recipient with reference to her bewitching features, while getting the colour of her eyes right, and not becoming too clinical about her other attractions.

Is it necessary for your poem to be witty as well? Here the Venetian versifier may be hard to emulate. The man could whip off a brilliant stanza at the drop of a hint. He left a trail of clever odes, as well as other babies, all across Europe, souvenirs that his lovers cherished long after he had waved goodbye.

What about the Casanovan's lifting his lyrical lines from a Hallmark greeting card? Hazardous, to say the least. It may not be a commercial crime, but plagiarism is bad for one's personal integrity. Surely it is better to lose one's love on the strength of one's own poems than to win her because she has been enchanted by a screed churned out by some hack Pindar in Peoria, Ill.

The composition of an *original* love poem begins with the purchase of a pencil (a slender length of lead encased in wood and topped with a vital eraser) and plenty of scrap paper. The Casanovan may even come to enjoy writing this way, steamy ballads that also seem to relieve his sinus problem.

[Note: do not e-mail your love poem. Some computers can't handle the divine afflatus.]

Pornography

". . . Whenever I see well-painted voluptuous pictures I feel myself on fire."

And Casanova had to depend on stills. Had he lived in our time of the X-rated porn film and the venereal video, he would have been chronically ablaze, to the point of incinerating himself.

As it was, denied these technological advances in depravity, he had to settle for paintings that had somehow not qualified for the Sistine Chapel. (Although the celebrated Ceiling does have some male nudes that turn on the more susceptible visitors.)

Casanova relied on his little boxed collection of obscene pictures, to share with ladies who needed to have their amatory pump primed . . .

"I took out a picture of a naked woman lying on her back and abusing herself . . . I shewed it to Leah."

Leah is not impressed. Laughs at the picture, in fact.

"No novelty for you?"

"Of course not. Every girl does like that before she gets married."

So much for pornography as a sure-fire stimulus for a woman. It appears that men are the more flammable gender, when it comes to naughty pictures. Women — who are all too likely to be RNs — take a more clinical interest in scenes of naked folk cavorting reproductively. They may, like Leah, just guffaw at the full monty.

The sad fact is that women are configured to look esthetically attractive in "voluptuous pictures," whereas men present a rather grotesque reminder that the beauty of nature sort of veers into burlesque, when the male mammal seeks to mount a charge.

Result: even in their raunchy novels, feminist authors' graphic descriptions of sex are couched in the context of romance.

Jacques, in contrast, could be aroused by the sight of a shapely bowl of fruit, if the banana was nestled between a couple of alluring melons. It was therefore a learning experience for him, as it will be for the Casanovan, that pornography has dubious value as an accelerant of women's libido. It appears to be less graceless when portrayed as homosexual intercourse of the lesbian ilk.

Of academic interest only, this, to the average guy. Who may safely assume that, mostly, porn is for . . . lorn.

☞ Positions

The apprentice Casanovan may need a special manual, to help with coupling of this order. Casanova himself, on occasion, as when pressed for time, found it expedient to provide his lover with graphic instructions for the assembly of various parts . . .

"Here is a small book which I have brought — the postures of

Pietro Aretino, which I want to try," he tells the adaptive nun Marie-Madeleine. Who demurs:

"But some of these poses could not be performed, and others are silly."

"True, but I have chosen four very interesting ones."

Apparently this workshop went well — ("These delightful labours occupied the remainder of the night") — but Casanova does not elaborate on the selected projects.

Pietro Aretino was born in 1492, the same year that another Italian explored regions of greater historical significance. His configuration surveys discovered nothing new, of course, as the classic 32 positions had long since been detailed by Greek, Roman, Arab and especially Hindu researchers, to say nothing of the Chinese, whose feats of acrobatics are legendary.

Most of these educational texts are less available than, say, the manual of instructions for connecting up one's VCR. Nearly all librarians are female. While they are apt to be more broad-minded than other curators of knowledge, the Casanovan will naturally hesitate to (a) cause the librarian undue amusement, or (b) arouse excessive cooperation.

Further, and as Casanova's nun sagely observed, some of the positions can be performed only by teenage gymnasts with rubber joints. The older Casanovan may not only fail to achieve the wild copulation attempted but could land up in Emergency as a human pretzel. Nurses and doctors can ask awkward questions, not adequately answered by his saying that he was attacked by a Murphy bed.

Also, as often happened with Jacques, when more than one woman is involved in this ecstatic mission, the positional combinations and permutations become exponentially complicated. He doesn't even attempt to describe the equivalent of the juggler's keeping ten plates spinning atop rods while he whistles "The Flight of the Bumblebee."

Some skills, alas, simply cannot be taught.

⇜ Possession

"What maintained my passion for Marie-Madeleine in a state of great vigour was that I never possessed her without running the risk of losing her."

Possession. A slippery noun. A man may possess a woman (in his own mind at least), or be possessed *with* a woman, or be possessed *by* a woman — all *bad* conditions, compared to the relatively benign state of possessing a Mickey Mouse watch.

If possessing nun Marie-Madeleine was a headache for Casanova — himself as easy to hold onto as a handful of mercury — no wonder the average guy today is apt to become even more antsy about his imagined ownership of a woman.

Only in football is possession more critical. Which may explain why so many men take refuge in stadium stands.

In the case of Giacomo's confused state of possession, the rival to whom he risked losing Marie-Madeleine was God. A formidable contender. In our time the competitive message is likely to come to our career woman via her beeper. Possibly while in bed. With the Casanovan *in extremis.*

Only the wealthy Greek ship owner, or Vegas gambling czar, can afford the bounteous blonde mistress who accepts the status of a possession, on threat of being suddenly retired into a dumpster.

Yet some oafs, under the delusion that they have sole and permanent possession of a woman, try to advertise this holding by:

1. putting their hat on her lap to show that she is taken.
2. wrapping an arm around her shoulders as if baling hay.
3. using the possessive pronoun "my" for other than their big mouth.

Possession may be nine-tenths of the law, but that remaining one-tenth makes a monkey of many a man. None of us is entirely immune to this dementia. The best advisory:

Be leery of any possession you can't get into a safety-deposit box.

≈ Pregnancy

Sex, basically, is a means of reproduction more pleasurable than Xeroxing. In Casanova's time — before invitro fertilization — it was the only means, a fact that rarely deterred him from unprotected intercourse. He was Mother Nature's plaything. But other mothers found him less amusing when their daughter started expanding at the waist.

Typically, Mme. Quinson, Jacques' landlady, gives him a hard time after her daughter Mimi fingers him as the producer of her enlargement. His counter-attack:

"How do you know that I am the father of the child?"

"Mimi says so. She is certain of it."

"I congratulate her, but I warn you, madame, that I am ready to swear that I have not any certainty about it."

Beautiful. A truly elegant parry of the blow. Not being threatened with a paternity suit based on DNA testing, Casanova could use that argument as unassailable. Which proves again that scientific progress is not an unadulterated blessing.

Another reason why the maestro rarely had to endure a scene with the outraged parent of a knocked-up lass: he never stayed as long as nine months in one town. By the time his work of helping to perpetuate the species became visible, he no longer was.

It should at once become apparent to the Casanovan that to remain as a permanent resident of a small town creates a sexual restraint second only to saltpetre, or marriage. It is no wonder that unwed mothers are less prevalent in the prairie village than in the big city, with ready access to an airport.

Being both promiscuous and peripatetic, Casanova created dozens of proud fathers, all over Europe, husbands who took credit for being the daddy of a son or daughter with fleeting resemblance, and the Casanova nose. Everyone was happy, and the population so buoyant as to barely notice attrition by war or plague.

So, "Are you on the pill, darling?" is a question no Casanovan should ever put to a woman he is bedding. Not only can it destroy a mood but it reflects a cautioned approach that most women find chilling. It doesn't pay to be too sensible with that sex. Never sacrifice passion to precaution, unless you are locked into a long-term lease of your apartment.

He who tries to think for both, ends up pleasing neither.

∽ Presumption

Don't count your chicks before they are laid.

Nothing can be more prejudicial to the success of a seduction than a man's coming across as fancying himself to be God's gift to women. A romantic legend in his own mind. In short, a dork.

Casanova never assumed. He had this rare talent: to be breathtakingly bold — his hands wee busier than a mute's at a garage sale — yet to somehow convey to the lady that her charms were so overwhelming that he had lost control of his libido.

He simply couldn't help himself. Except to her.

An example of gross presumption is the behaviour of the guy who sidles up to the prettiest woman sitting at the bar and, winking, asks "Do you wanna f—?" Women have nothing but contempt for men who leave out the last letters of a word, for fear of offending.

Also an error: leering. Casanova never leered. Or ogled. Or made kissy noises with his lips. He kept his entire face under control, letting his eyes do the talking. His eyes did *not* say "Here I am, you lucky broad, and I know you want me right now." With Giacomo, the gaze was penetrating yet not presumptuous.

Some Casanovans find it difficult to lock looks with a handsome woman and talk at the same time. This is why it helps to hold a glass of wine, to occupy the mouth while you concentrate on your forthright regard. If the wine spills, it spills.

At least you will have left the presuming to Stanley, staring at Dr. Livingstone.

∽ Principles

Was Casanova totally unprincipled? Morally underprivileged? Not the ideal role model for the young man eager to qualify for sainthood?

Well, possibly. But he does offer his memoirs as a cautionary tale for the parents of daughters. He trusts that the accounts of his "amorous exploits" will alert them to other, less principled lovers, who may debauch young women without loving them as he did, in his uniquely compensatory way.

However, and though no statistics are available, it seems fair to say that Casanova's memoirs have not found a place in the family library, beside The Holy Bible, Dr. Spock and *Nanook of the North*.

The reason for its glaring absence — aside from the fact that the multiple volumes take up more shelf space than Mom cares to dust — may be that it is hard to identify exactly what Casanova is warning parents against. After all, his guiding principle during his travels was that he was a sort of missionary, whose sole, dedicated service was that of giving pleasure to women and taking it, in equal measure.

This was his concept of equal gender rights. And the doctrine certainly makes rosier reading than anything issued from the Friedans and Milletts, till Phase Two, The Big Ahem.

For this reason, the Casanovan should not be overly influenced by a mea culpa with whiskers on it. Or, if he wishes to cover all the bases of principled conduct, he can give his girl-friend a copy of Casanova's memoirs (abridged edition) as a Christmas present. Then she will be aware that his dating her goes beyond escorting her to a Disney movie.

No, Jacques Casanova was not a knight in shining armour. He didn't even have a good relationship with horses. For what he sought to mount, horse and helmet were both supernumerary. On principle.

∽ Promiscuity

At one point in his financial career, Casanova owned a silk factory that employed "a score of girls, nearly all of them pretty and seductive, as most Parisienne girls are . . . a reef on which my virtue was shipwrecked every day."

Giacomo's virtue was a rather frail craft to start with. Being the boss of a "score" (what else?) of females eager to get on in industry, he was in no wise caulked against temptation . . .

"My fancy never lasted more than a week, and often waned in three or four days, and the latest comer always appeared the most worthy of my attention."

As the tone of this report suggests, Casanova didn't really feel challenged by this supervision of his all-girl staff. It was assembly-line sex. No craftsmanship required. Also, business was bad. The whole, brief factory episode proved to be something of an aberration, in his relations with women.

So, should Casanova be labeled as sexually promiscuous? No. What Casanova was, was socially active.

Every woman he had was the *only* woman in his life, though their affair might last only a week or so. The point is that he gave more of himself to the love of the moment, in whatever length of time, than most men can summon in a relationship that lasts longer than either partner cares to remember.

Promiscuity is determined by the relativity of time. More, the promiscuous person may simply be incapable of love, emotionally sterile. The Casanovan, in contrast, will emulate his idol by throwing his heart recklessly into every affair, regardless of his need to catch a plane or attend his grandmother's funeral.

What the judgmental see as promiscuity may truly be viewed as the variety that is the spice of life. And who of us would choose a bland existence, over the Italian's peppery pizza of a lifestyle?

≈ Prostate

Fittingly, a sex gland was the death of the world's greatest lover. Casanova died, at seventy-three, of a diseased prostate. Cause: probably the other big C. Even so, he lived to a remarkably old age, in a century when people were fortunate to hit fifty. Much credit must be given to his dedication to a regime of aerobic exercise that required no equipment other than a sturdy bed, and of course a pretty woman.

The young Casanovan is apt to give little or no thought to his prostate. He may even refer to it as his "prostrate" — a favourite position rather than the walnut-sized generator of seminal fluid and maker of life miserable in later years.

His enlarged prostate (benign prostatic hyperplasia) will interfere with the sex life of the older Casanovan by clamping the urethra (pee-way) and creating the frequent, urgent calls of nature that ruin a romantic tryst anywhere farther than 100 feet from a W.C. Yet urologists recommend regular ejaculation to minimize the colonizing of bad bugs in the prostate.

No, this is not a heroic measure.

What *does* require a stiffening of the upper lip — and is the measure that might have prolonged Casanova's life — is the rectal examination to probe the prostate for suspicious bumps and lumps that presage cancer.

It is hard to imagine the cocky Casanovan submitting to this digital survey, unless it was performed by a female physician . . . in a candlelit examining room . . . with naughty pictures on the walls.

As for prostatitits, if the Casanovan has reason to believe that he has been cursed with this malady — which can affect men of any age and make the Grand Canyon look like minor depression — he definitely should *not* have sex with a woman he loves.

Bite the bullet and keep the bugs to yourself. Thus making the grade as a martyr as unsung as any never recorded.

❧ Quid Pro Quo

"All women, dear Leah, whether they are honest or not, are for sale. When a man has plenty of time he buys the woman his heart desires by unremitting attentions; but when he's in a hurry he buys her with presents, and even with money."

Which of course explains why rich men have the prettiest wives and girlfriends. They can afford to be in a hurry. While the poor man has to soldier on with "unremitting attentions" and no guarantee that the sale will be finalized in his lifetime.

Casanova had both money and time enough to purchase the pleasure of having any woman he wanted. He had the capacity to accelerate his attentions, so that a woman had been bought before she even realized that she was on special.

However, the Casanovan who assumes that he can have any woman he craves, simply on the strength of his physique and personal charm, may be fantasizing. True, today's gender equality has, for him, changed the criteria for buy and sell. There is always the chance that he will meet a lovely female who has the means to buy him, for *her* sexual gratification. He shouldn't quibble. But, usually he is not the main reason why women go to the mall.

For the Casanovan as for the Master, sex with a woman is never a freebie. The cost will vary, from a case of beer to a case of child support. But the bottom line is inexorable: something for nothing exists only in his dreams.

Once the Casanovan accepts that fact of love life, he can go shopping for a woman with the same sensible zest with which she shops for a pair of shoes. Expect to pay more than you can afford, in both time and coin of the realm. But never doubt that the quo is well worth the quid.

∾ Rationale

Giacomo, at eighteen, gets the toothsome fourteen-year old Lucie in trouble by not going all the way with her. He blames himself for his self-restraint. If he had yielded totally to desire, he says, "she would not have been left by me in that state of ardent excitement . . . she would not have fallen prey to that scoundrel." (Lucie runs away from home with a callous postal courier who gets her pregnant and abandons her.)

Stricken with guilt, the young Casanova vowed, "I would never again remain uncertain and timid where love and my partner urged me on." That he stayed resolutely true to that pledge is one of the great inspirational messages of the memoirs.

For the rest of a long and sexually active life, Casanova dedicated himself to ensuring that no woman he rogered was other than completely satisfied. He guaranteed that there was no chance that she would ever fall victim to another man simply because Casanova had broken the egg without making the omelette.

A public service. That is the way — rather than mock it as a rationale — to describe this lay saint's determination to free his love affairs from any goal but total gratification, to go forth boldly where no man had gone before, let alone followed.

The Casanova disciple must therefore overcome his natural deference and timidity, remembering that the more pleasure he gives the maiden in bringing her to multiple orgasm, the greater his contribution to social welfare.

It may be argued that Casanova was merely rationalizing, finding an excuse for never being satisfied with a kiss on the cheek. Question is: was it a rationale that rendered him unforgettable to so many women?

Remember: "The heart has its reasons, which the mind knows nothing of." (Pascal, bless him.)

Reciprocity

"The happiness I gave her increased mine twofold, for it has always been my weakness to receive half of my enjoyment from the happiness which I give to my charming partner."

As our mother used to tell us: it's nice to share.

In pornographic film studios the key to reciprocated sex is known as "getting her hot." Which can take longer than, say, shooting the collision of two automobiles.

The young Casanovan, in his precipitate assault, is apt to forget that a groan from his partner is not necessarily a compliment to his performance. A woman will shout "Yes! Yes! Yes!" in order to get something over with. Also known as "faking it."

Did Casanova ever have a woman fake her enjoyment of their intercourse? Probably. But the exception was so rare that one searches the thousands of pages of his memoirs in vain, to find a reference to his even suspecting that his partner's response was mere sound effects.

But he does acknowledge that his close — very close — attention to the woman's pleasure was "my weakness." His raising love-making to an art cost him a lot of time and physical effort. (A guy can easily dislocate an elbow.) And it was his pride as a virtuoso that pushed him to satisfy the lady as well as his basic, animal urge to procreate. He distanced himself from rape as far as possible, unless we consider wine to have an unfair influence on a woman's will-power.

Such noble endeavour raises reciprocity beyond the word's usual connotation of commerce between countries. It makes the World Trade Organization look relatively tawdry. Much more contented would be at least half the world's population — the female half — if all men honoured the ideal of reciprocity as conceived by Jacques Casanova.

❧ Regret

"I looked back upon my life and did not like what had become of me. Where was the man I had been, a gentler man, a more constant one, perhaps a more honest man."

Yes, Casanova too had his mid-life crisis. He managed to hold it off till he was pretty old, but he could not escape the account sheet of a life based on libertinism, as a religious faith.

The Casanovan too should be prepared to cope with the universal regret of every sexually active man: that he let get away the girl who really mattered. With Casanova, it was Tonine . . . "and what embitters my old age is that, having a heart as warm as ever, I have no longer the strength necessary to secure a single day as blissful as those which I owed to this charming girl."

The man who, later in life, has nothing to regret probably has little worth remembering. Old men draw strength mostly from their memories. These provide cold comfort if they include no Tonine, or Henriette, or any of dozens of other loving women.

Casanova never regretted what he had done, only that he had become too pooped to perpetuate it.

The Casanovan should also remember that Jacques' main regret was not his love life but the attendant squandering of his other resources, with the result that he entered old age not only alone but poverty-stricken. The old adage — "whom the gods love die young" — applies most pertinently to adventurers like our Venetian playboy. The gods, obviously, didn't love him half as well as did much of the female population of continental Europe.

However, the Casanovan whose first thought is to avoid doing anything that he may later regret is likely to be frozen into a state of sexual stasis. He may desert the whole lifestyle, taking refuge in marriage and a balanced mutual fund. Both of which bear the potential of other regrets, which mature much earlier than those that afflicted our wizard of wooing.

Regret is part of the package we call life. The trick is to delay feeling it, for as long as possible, with the diversion of the daily round of golf that combines regrets with a bit of exercise.

⟐ Rejection

Rejection by a woman is the hardest kind of straight-arm that a Casanovan can suffer. Much more painful, this is, than rejection by, say, an army recruiting office, or by a motor-vehicle branch driver's test.

Casanova, though rarely thus rejected by a woman he desired, was devastated when the disaster did occur . . .

"For two hours after" (learning that the lovely Manon would be marrying someone else) "I was bereft of my senses. I wrote and tore up scores of letters, a thousand designs came to my disordered imagination. I spent that day and the night that followed in delirious thoughts. *Now I see that my self-love and vanity were outraged, but then I was ill and hurt.*" (Italics added)

Every Casanovan should adopt that last sentence as his mantra.

If he also strikes a gong, while mumbling it, that is better than hitting his head against the wall. A man whose amatory hopes have been rebuffed can become a dangerous object, one that should be kept locked up till his ego stops whining.

With Casanova, the suicidal impulse was short-lived. In the sad case of La Charpillon, the gorgeous London whore who trifled bigtime with his affection, he expedited his recovery by buying a parrot that he trained to squawk "Miss Charpillon is a bigger tart than her mother." He put the parrot up for sale, guaranteeing that enough people would hear the message to spread it abroad. The victim's lawyers were thwarted because "a parrot cannot be indicted for libel."

Today, not only are parrots more expensive to buy, but the whole concept of revenge as therapy for rejection is not viable. "Stalking" — a common resort of the rejected lover — is now a criminal offense. It is a serious mistake even to be seen in the same neighborhood, if not the same town, as a woman on the alert for a stalking lover.

Casanova usually shortened his misery by getting out of town altogether. The old amour-propre recovers faster with a change of scene, where the Casanovan can see more clearly that he was rejected because the unfortunate woman is:

1. a latent lesbian, or
2. really, really frigid, or
3. a man-eating psychopath, or
4. from Toronto.

Or, of course, all of the above.

~ Reputation

Then as now, a man's having a reputation as a charming rogue drew women more surely than his being known as a living saint.

Thus Casanova enjoyed the spinoff from two personal records, one his high percentage of hits on women, the other his being clapped into, and dramatic escape from, The Leads prison in Venice. (He wrote a book about the latter caper, a best-seller throughout Europe and precursor of today's vogue of the published works of both male and female ex-cons.)

In fisherman's terms, Casanova had the reputation of The Big One That Got Away. A lure for women who are not often found at the end of a conventional rod because their angling is to catch a guy. And the challenge of shooting fish in a barrel does not excite them as much as that of hooking — even briefly — the social swim's Moby Dick.

This does *not* mean that the Casanovan should pass himself off as a notorious scofflaw and seducer when he has done nothing to deserve the reputation. Yet he does need to convey that he is not just a clean-living chap, with no record of breaking out of jail or into women.

He must strive for a lurid, sex-charged reputation that no one can verify. Difficult, yes. Even if he bears a passing resemblance to Mick Jagger.

This may require moving to another country. Don't pack the sincere tie.

⁓ Resistance

"I kissed with rapture her beautiful hands, but she thought fit to pose some resistance. Oh, how sweet they are, those denials of a loving mistress who delays the happy moment only for the sake of enjoying its delights better!"

Easy victories are not as memorable. Every Casanovan faces the daunting fact: a woman will resent him for testing her resistance, and despise him for not doing so. Casanova himself was confused about this paradox, writing elsewhere in his memoirs:

"Those who prefer a little resistance to an easy conquest are in the wrong; but a too easy conquest often points to a depraved nature, and this men do not like, however depraved they themselves may be."

Casanova was often able to overcome his dislike of depravity, if he was in a hurry to leave town anyhow. But the relatively static Casanovan may have his judgment, and timing, severely tried by his date's resistance. "Three dates and you're in" — the current timetable for compliance — is not altogether foolproof, if the lady is not counting.

Although Casanova's own life may be described as one long romp down the garden path of least resistance, his opportunities to freewheel were more apparent than such are to men today.

Their recognizing their inability to measure units of resistance in the feminist disposition is why some men take the easy way out of such physics: the hooker. But it is with that gorgeous yet somehow forbidding Ms. Maybe in Shipping that the Casanovan must feel his way without rubber gloves.

He may be comforted by the admission of the consummate swain: ". . . I possessed myself of the most beautiful bosom, which I smothered under my kisses. But her favours went no further, and I doubled my efforts in vain."

As Lincoln's Union troops discovered: the more one closes in on the South, the stiffer the resistance becomes. Pray for victory, but anticipate defeat.

◈ Restraint

"Yet I thought it would be good policy to appear ignorant of her inclination for me, and to let her suppose . . . that I was in love with her, but that my love appeared hopeless. I knew that such a plan was infallible, because it saved her dignity."

Casanova here is maneuvering against the beautiful marchioness friend of a powerful cardinal of Rome. But his strategy applies to any woman in a position to expect a restrained approach: female business executive, university professor (women's studies), police sergeant, flight attendant (over 30 thousand feet), coroner . . . any of whom may appear extremely attractive to a sensual man with a short fuse.

His restraint must not be based on appearances. The one thing that the modern woman's swimsuit does not reveal is her dignity. Which can turn a normal, healthy impulse into an arrest for assault.

Casanova, however, knew the value of restraint. By behaving as though he assumed that his love for the marchioness was hopeless, he showed the deference that he knew to be pure catnip for even the most top-bred pussies.

He let his eyes do the talking, while his tongue watched its step and his hands took early retirement.

Thus he cues the Casanovan who, though not likely to encounter many marchionesses at the bowling alley, will be more likely to impress favourably the contemporary lady if:

1. he restrains his admiring gaze from taking up residency in her cleavage.

2. he refrains from expressing his admiration by (a) whistling, (b) drumming the feet on the ground, (c) drooling.
3. he doesn't try to kiss her in public, unless celebrating the end of World War II.

↝ Rule #1

"We" (Casanova added Thérèse, another teenager guesting at dinner in a senator's home) "were sitting down at a table very near each other, our backs to the door of the room in which we thought our patron fast asleep. Somehow we took a fancy to examine the difference of conformation between a girl and boy. But at the most interesting moment of our study, a violent blow on my shoulders from a stick, followed by another, and which would be followed by many more if I had not run away, compelled me to abandon our interesting investigation, unfinished."

The caning "rapped a message into my skull which I read to mean 'Never get caught!' And that message is one which in the years that followed I seldom if ever forgot."

Luckily for posterity, Giacomo did not let this doctrine impede his continued research into female anatomy. He just never turned his back on a sleeping patron. He also was enormously lucky in rarely getting caught with his pants down and the contents up.

He usually put a fair amount of planning into his conquests, though the several times when he conducted his investigation while riding in a carriage or gondola may encourage the Casanovan to translate the exploration site into today's transportation. Resulting perhaps in being charged with more than a traffic violation.

Getting caught in the act by a cop can be psychologically damaging, to the point of one's being rendered impotent, for as long as a week.

The threat of being caught is one good reason for having reasonably private accommodation, for sex, rather than the public beach, golf course or back row of the cinema.

⌁ Satan

Casanova's landlady has sent her nubile and (literally) fetching daughter, Tonine, to wait on him at supper. He is at once beguiled by the fifteen-year-old's budding charms. In the spirit of good fellowship (he tells himself), he invites the teenager to dine with him . . .

"I did everything in good faith. By and by, reader, we shall see whether this is not one of the devices by which the Devil composes his ends."

Get thee behind me, Satan — and push!

In Casanova's era, despite its being the Age of Enlightenment, the Devil was still being given his due, for corrupting the good intentions of a decent gentleman in the presence of a dishy young lady. Giacomo provided the Prince of Darkness with a favourite target for turning good faith into naughty fact.

Of the seven deadly sins, the only one that he didn't give a good workout was sloth. Lust, anger, gluttony, envy, pride and covetousness he excelled in. But he was never lazy. He was "always on the job," as the English say. Busy enough to reduce the hounds of Hell to whimpering curs.

The Casanovan of today may have more difficulty in claiming that, as a chronic womanizer, he is the victim of Mephisto's wiles.

When his soul arrives at the Pearly Gate, and St. Peter merely raises an eyebrow by way of reception, he likely will plead that his spirit was subverted by TV commercials.

The man himself never let fear of the Devil impede the even stronger power of Desire. It took only a little seductive encouragement from Tonine, wearing a smock too brief in all directions, to make him surrender to Satan — "the die was cast." And so Caesar "had an exquisite dinner which my charming Tonine prepared, served and shared with me. Looking at her as at the same time my wife, my mistress and my house-keeper, I was delighted to find myself so happy at such a cheap rate."

Rates have gone up, obviously, along with hems. The Casanovan must decide for himself, case by case, to what extent he is being made the pawn of Auld Hornie, or just Fredericks of Hollywood.

⌇ Satyriasis

Did Casanova suffer from a slight case of satyriasis?

Some of the symptoms are evident in the memoirs:

– a sexual arousal time measured in nanoseconds

– a willingness to risk all the less central parts of his body, in order to satisfy a need not normally considered to be life threatening

– a very restricted view of cardio-vascular exercise

– a one-track mind with no crossing signal.

Casanova often complains, in his writings, about this sexual compulsion that cost him so much time and money, as well as several painful episodes of lecher's plague. But he obviously learned to live with his affliction which, mercifully, is one of the few conditions that lessen as a person gets older.

How does a man distinguish between satyriasis and just having a normal urge to screw every attractive woman he meets? Certainly Jacques did not fit the description of the randy faun — short, fuzzy ears, twitchy tail, etc. — but the Casanovan who notices horns budding on his brow may be wise to have his doctor check him out for goat breath.

Casanova does not seem to have seen himself as being hyper-lustful. He always thought that he had just fallen in love, again, very, very quickly. And few of the women causing this sudden descent into *amore* questioned the logistics. Such is the vanity of a beautiful young girl that she expects instant devotion, which just happens to coincide with the guy's grabbing her fanny.

The best way to quell qualms about being a suppressed satyr is to remember that male urologists agree: sex is healthful. Unless of course the lady has a husband. In which case your physical status can decline suddenly.

➡ Seduction

To Casanova, it was a dirty word. Seduction meant something that other libertines did to women, i.e. not cricket. Thus when he meets his beloved Marie-Madeleine #2, he finds her already pregnant by "her seducer, a monster called M. de Coudet."

Or, he will deal with seduction as an abstract concept, a generalized process: "If the seducer is clever the young innocent will soon have gone too far to draw back . . ."

It is the difference between describing how to make a bomb and actually throwing one.

That Casanova himself was frequently the victim of seduction (by women) is abundantly clear to anyone reading his memoirs. Belatedly, he admitted that he had been duped with the regularity of Greenwich time, but he was having too good a time to realize that he had been had.

Hopeless romantic that he was, our genial Giacomo didn't think of sexual involvement with a woman as other than the fortuitous collision of heavenly bodies. That was his universe. He didn't care whether it was planned by God or the laws of chance. Intercourse was something that happened, not planned.

Those of us who, unfortunately, have more opportunity to be objective can judge that Casanova was guilty of seducing more than the legal limit of very young girls. In our time the law would have him by the short and curlies, and no fun at all.

⮞ Sex

". . . that sex without which man would be the most miserable animal on earth."

Casanova here uses the word "sex" in the only sense he ever does so, namely as *gender*. As in "the fair sex." Never does he describe amatory endeavour as "having sex" with a woman. To do so would cheapen the entire exercise, which in Casanova's judgment was his finest hour. If not longer.

He would have been disgusted by the verbal debasement of love-making familiar to us of coarser tongue. *Screwing*, for instance, does not occur on any page of the thousands that he wrote. As for the f-word — his quill would have moulted.

Casanova had only one word [*see* LOVE] for the physical manifestation of his enchantment by the opposite sex. For him, the experience provided much more than release from sexual tension. The female sex rescued him, and other men of otherwise sound mind, from being "the most miserable animal on earth."

Woody Allen — master of the miserable — captures the contemporary status of sex in a memorable bit of dialogue in his *Love and Death* . . .

Sonja: Oh, don't Boris! Please! Sex without love is an empty experience.

Boris: Yes, but — as empty experiences go — it's one of the best!

To Casanova — as it should be to Everyman — making love to a woman is ennobling. A refining of raw libido. Wooing a beautiful woman brought out the best in him, as it has done from Pindar (odes) to Shakespeare (sonnets) to Gershwin (melodies).

One of the sad effects of the alienation of the genders — a plague upon the 21st century — is that men are foregoing that transmutation from brute to something better. The quick fix of pornography has replaced the sensitive arts with which Casanova captivated women of every age and social station.

Worse, many women too are reduced to miserable creatures, whining their way into the week's Top Ten Bleats.

Can the disciple restore some to the magic? Not for all western society, perhaps, but for himself it's a worthy goal. Most women still respond favourably to being treated as a different, and esteemed, sex. And will bring to love-making their inimitable stimulus to the finer sentiments in both partners.

A chorus, gentlemen, of "There's Nothing Like a Dame!"

✎ Sleep

"We abandoned ourselves to love, then to sleep, then to love again and so on alternately till daybreak."

Casanova was a firm believer in the value of sleep. Alternately. This behavioral pattern undoubtedly contributed to his stamina, as a sexual prodigy. While he frequently, and because of special circumstances like those imposed by his banging the wife of his prison's governor, would settle for what we now call "a quickie," he understood that sleeping with a woman meant just that: an interval of contiguous slumber that extended his eternal devotion to last at least overnight.

He also understood that a gentleman always lets his lover fall asleep first. The most unpardonable sin, in bed, is for the man to satisfy himself hurriedly, then lapse into snoring oblivion, regardless of the fact that a woman takes longer to become sexually sated.

Too, Casanova adapted readily to sleeping in a strange bed. Indeed, his bed was rarely as familiar as the woman he had in it. The Casanovan may find that his sex drive is compromised by a bumpy mattress, or alien bed-springs that seem to be squeaking "Tsk! Tsk!" If so, he should take conditioning training in BEDS, sleeping alone in second-rate motels till he is distracted by nothing short of a major earthquake.

The act of sleeping together, after sex, provides the special bonding of lovers that is denied to couples who have it off during their lunch-break.

What of the woman who falls asleep before the Casanovan has consummated this tender union? Not to worry! It happened to

Giacomo, too, though not often. He blamed it on the wine, counted on her sweet dreams, continued with his caresses . . . "and when at last I abandoned myself to all the force of passion, she awoke with a sigh of bliss, murmuring 'Ah! It is true then!'"

Sleep not only "knitteth up the ravelled sleeve of care" but doth a lot of other restorative work. And the arms of Morpheus are of N.B.A.-length enough to embrace both lovers.

⌇ Soliloquy

"To be, or not to be . . ." There will be times when the Casanovan, too, feels suicidal. Because of a woman.

It may be some comfort to know that Casanova himself, despite his stunning track record and resilient nature, could be moved to an impassioned soliloquy that makes Hamlet look dumbfounded.

When stricken by "conflicting feelings of love, surprise and uncertainty," he confesses to us, "I must speak aloud, and I throw so much action, so much animation, into these monologues that I forget that I am alone."

Speaking to the walls, as he did, is not much recognized today as effective catharsis. Women have the advantage of talking to other women, or a psychologist. But a man usually balks at blabbing his woe to others unless too drunk to remember what was said. He bottles it up. This pressurizes stress to the detriment of all the vital organs, and can also affect his driving. Much of the road rage that we observe on the highway derives from some guy's pent-up frustration with a woman.

If the Casanovan is living at home, with family or pets that are already nervous, his soliloquizing may be inhibited. Especially if, like Jacques, he accompanies the discourse with "action" and "animation." It may be necessary to rent a room somewhere, or hike a fair distance into the woods, in order to give full, active expression to his angst.

Does the monologue solve the problem? Unfortunately, no. As Casanova admits, "it made me still more angry." Sooner or later it is necessary to confront something more responsive that the bathroom door. I.e., the maddening Ms.

But the lover's soliloquy may provide the benefit of focusing his fury. The Casanovan will, with luck, have eliminated the more irrational elements of his tirade. He may also be induced to keep his voice down, if neighbours complain to police.

Silence is golden, but it won't buy peace of mind. That is why God created beer.

➤ Stamina

"Zenobia, in the flower of youth, reached heaven many more times than I did. Just as I lost life for the third time and Zenobia for the fourteenth, I heard visitors and we dressed hastily."

By his own admission, Casanova was a sexual athlete of Olympian class. With the magnificent and challenging Madeleine, he pushes the record to new heights . . .

". . . during seven hours I gave her the most positive proof of my ardour and the feelings I entertained for her . . . I varied our pleasures in a thousand different ways, and I astonished her by making her feel that she was susceptible of greater enjoyment than she had any idea of . . ."

Sobering stats, these, for the amateur Casanovan. What strikes us other mere mortals is Casanova's meticulous record of these statistics, recalled years later for his memoirs. Did he keep a score sheet, updated regularly? Or did he just have a remarkable memory for outstanding performances, like the commentators on Monday Night Football?

That Casanova was not on steroids is obvious. The sort of performance at which he excelled, and which won the silent applause of hundreds of women, depends on a physical endowment that owes nothing to a high-fibre diet or drinking eight glasses of water a day.

Casanova prided himself on inducing climax in his partner more times than he came himself. That requires a certain standard of dedication. In scoring assists to goals, this man was the Wayne Gretzky of womanizers.

Should the Casanovan be discouraged if he fails to achieve such feats of endurance? Well, probably. But not to the point of taking early retirement from his career as a lover. By concentrating on the pleasure he is giving a woman, and finding innovative ways to drive her crazy, he will learn the secret of all great athletes: *pacing*.

Pacing is something that a man will never develop by having it off in the back seat of a car, or in the office elevator, or some other travesty of Casanovism. It betrays an interest in other activities. And fails to build stamina, the difference between a single-shot pistol and the veritable Uzi automatic that was Jacques Casanova.

STD

As might be expected, our Seigneur de Seingalt had several run-ins with sexually transmitted disease, which he never identified in his memoirs as other than a totally unwarranted disaster . . .

"My assassin was La Renard. I cannot imagine what had become of my wits to let myself be so beguiled, while every day I renewed the poison that this serpent poured into my veins . . . I was almost killed by a clumsy doctor before I was cured of the present this vixen had bestowed on me . . ."

Casanova received at least four such little gratuitous gifts during his life. Each time he expresses the same surprise and outrage . . .

". . . I met an attractive young governess, Maton, who was seeking employment, which I immediately gave her, and then was off to Dresden with my governess. I saw signs that she was willing to exchange favors with the young officers who frequented our inn, but she denied this. Then I discovered that this innocent-looking monster had infected me, and also poisoned the military gallants . . ."

So much for relying on an employee's resumé.

The only medical treatment for VD in Casanova's time was a topical application of mercury compound, an operation performed without anaesthetic, though the patient might die of embarrassment. Mercury, one of the least likable of metallic elements, should never be let out of the thermometer or barometer, to tussle with bugs on one's prize bloomer.

Today's treatment relies on less brutal antibiotics, but come-uppance has kept pace with the emergence of AIDS. Thus the Casanovan lives under the reign of terror that is the CONDOM — both male and female formats . . . Hark! The squeak of rubber on rubber! If music be the food of love, here's strange obbligato!

Yet, prudence rules. That old alibi — "I must have picked it up in a toilet on the ferry" — nice try, but no cigar. Unless the Casanovan has taken up permanent residence in a public lavatory, slim and none are the chances of being infected by the jakes. The john who preceded you at a massage parlour, yes, he might be the source of your affliction. But an act of God, it probably ain't.

The Casanovan will do well to remember actor Peter Lorre's wonderful line in *The Maltese Falcon,* when he is hoisted aloft by the hulking Sydney Greenstreet:

"Put me down! You don't know where I've been!"

Indeed we don't, ma'am.

➣ Suicide

"In despair I made my way to Westminster Bridge with the intention of leaping to my death."

Here Casanova is reporting on his parlous state of mind after being frustrated by the harlot Charpillon. Definitely not the highlight of his visit to London, this gorgeous tramp pushed all his buttons. Yet it was a mature womanizer she was dealing with, not some downy-cheeked lad sans an impressive *curriculum vitae* of sexual conquest to bolster his self-esteem.

In the event, the desperate Jacques was deterred from polluting the Thames with his corpse, by a friendly passerby, an Englishman kind enough to take him to a nearby pub. Else the memoirs might never have been written, and mankind denied the great testament to carnal relations.

The Casanovan may smile at the master's over-reaction to REJEC-TION. But he should never underestimate the power of a woman to put his ego through the shredder. She need not be a prostitute to take pleasure in his misery. The feminist movement has generated a plethora of mean-spirited game-players, whose main delight is to render some simple, one-track-minded guy ready to kill himself.

To be treated so may not drive the Casanovan to contemplate suicide, but it certainly will not help him to quit smoking, or drinking, or driving through red lights.

Joining a private golf club that excludes women does provide some relief for the thwarted lover, by replacing one extreme frustration with a bigger one.

Very expensive, however. Even if the Casanovan is playing with used golfballs, it is less costly to avoid the man-eater by other means.

Do *not* frequent singles bars. These are where lurk the truly brassed-off dames whose pastime it is to give a randy man good reason to slash his wrists.

And one should try to see such women objectively, as suffering from loss of innocence. *"Tout comprendre, c'est tout pardonner."* To understand everything, is to forgive everything. And, besides, jumping off a bridge, into a river, can draw a nasty letter from Greenpeace.

∽ Temptation

"I can resist anything but temptation" — the Wilde mantra of the flamboyantly feeble-willed.

Was Casanova ever subject to the temptation that would have destroyed his career and reputation as the man who made Cupid's arrows fly like Henry's at Agincourt? Namely, the temptation to give up his peripatetic pursuit of pleasure, mostly in the form of pulchritudinous popsies? To retire to a cozy cottage, with a devoted mortgage? Shuck the dancing shoes in favour of slippers under the marital bed? The promiscuous lips stilled by a briar pipe, the ogling eyes blinkered by family responsibilities, and his roving restricted to walking the poodle?

Well, no. According to his memoirs, Casanova was tempted (by MARRIAGE) once or twice. But always with women who were unlikely to accept a proposal, because either they were already married or engaged, or they were shrewd enough to recognize that being wed to Giacomo Casanova would be like trying to grasp quicksilver.

Lacking the master's sublime dedication to dalliance, the Casanovan is more likely to yield to the temptation to settle down with one woman, or another guy, or a female cat with some sense of loyalty. It is a lure — domesticity — that gets stronger with each passing airline meal.

But at least he can try to fend off the temptation as long as possible, like a goalie in the NHL playoff. If he makes it past forty, he deserves appointment to The Sports Hall of Ill Fame. After fifty, the Order of Casanova Medal. With fig leaf.

∼ Termination

Casanova's conscience was splendidly clear, with regard to getting a woman pregnant. This because he had already blown the burg before she realized that his seed had been firmly planted.

Usually the first inkling he had that he had effected conception was when he visited the same town many years later, and was introduced to an adolescent son or daughter, by a mother who was delighted to repeat her blunder.

Occasionally, however, Casanova would take a fancy to a pretty girl who was gravid by someone else, and who was desperate to terminate the incubation of a bastard. Ever the opportunist when attracted to a maiden in distress, Jacques persuades the fair Guistiniana to try a remedy recommended by his daffy sponsor, Mme. d'Urfé: the Aroph of Paracelsus. Easy to apply — with "a cylindrical instrument of sufficient size and length" — the probe is anointed at the tip with an unguent of saffron, virgin honey, and any other condiments that come to hand at short notice.

The dose has to be repeated several times a day, for a week, but satisfaction is guaranteed. No abortion, perhaps, but a great emotional release . . .

"We looked solemn — I was a medical student about to perform an operation, she like the patient, and also the nurse who makes ready the instruments. Then we set about the operation, both as grave as two doctors of divinity . . ."

Never one to leave the outcome in doubt, Casanova repeats the operation many times over the course of a week, pausing only to sleep and reload the therapeutic cylinder.

And the patient thrives on the treatment. As Casanova enjoys his dedication to his practice: "Though I was in love with this charming girl, I did not feel in the least ashamed of having deceived her, especially as what I did could have no adverse effect." And how many other gynecologists can make that statement?

In the end, Jacques arranges for Guistiniana to find refuge in a convent, "where she remained until delivered of a fine boy." And how many convents today offer this facility?

Abortion on demand — the latest nostrum for unwanted pregnancy — limits the chance that Dr. Casanovan can be of such service. Wearing a stethoscope around your neck may impress a few women, but the thing *can* dangle in your latté.

～ Theatre

"I was chiefly interested in kept women, and those of the theatre. The halls of the theatres are capital places for amateurs to exercise their talent in intrigue, and I profited by the lessons I learned in this fine school."

So sayeth the young theatre critic.

As a prime source of compliant lovers, the theatre provided Giacomo with women as (a) actresses and/ or dancers, (b) those in "boxes occupied only by pretty women." He also, of course, being a very able and successful dramatist himself, was sometimes interested in what was occurring on the stage in terms of a theatrical production. But if the play or ballet happened to be worth his attention, that was just a bonus.

Casanova didn't need a program, to make eye contact with the bosomy belle fluttering her fan in the box. Often there was more high drama developing in the loges than on the stage: the first act of a sex play whose dénouement would be set in Casanova's sack.

Comely women who receive mass adoration can afford to be less concerned about commitment. Also, since his actresses were as peripatetic as Casanova himself, their moral status was free of the scrutiny of a community.

Conclusion: attending live theatre can be an excellent social resource for the Casanovan who has scruples about skiing.

Unfortunately, the small, intimate theatre of Casanova's time — romantically aglow with candles or lamps, plushy in the velvet of the private boxes — has largely disappeared. It is hard to make eye contact with a woman in the Ford Centre for the Performing Arts. Without using binoculars, that is.

Still, as a venue for flirting, the theatre should be seriously considered by the amateur Casanovan who has drawn a blank at the Boston Marathon. This despite the low-percentage chance of his getting a shot at a member of the chorus line of *Cats*.

Attending the theatre remains a viable alternative to depending upon his computer's chat-line, putting himself at the mercy of a mouse. The woman in the flesh is to be trusted better than a talking head, with its terrifying potential for disillusionment when one actually meets the feet.

[Note: most fringe theatres now cater largely to gays and lesbians. Wrong scene.]

⁓ Therapy

One of Casanova's many talents was his skill as an unlicensed physician. He brought colour to the cheeks of several lovelies who appeared to be hovering at death's door. There is no record of his ever having cured a man of a complaint, except by running him through with his sword. And there was a certain sameness about the therapy that he provided for pale virgins, pregnant spinsters and other women who had not responded to being bled.

In essence, Casanova's was a heat treatment . . .

". . . after her eating dinner with me, we went to my balcony where I made her share in the fire which consumed me. As I pressed her lovingly to my bosom she completed my bliss with such warmth that I could see that she thought she was receiving a favour and not granting one."

Medicare, eat your heart out!

The healing power of good sex has long had its place in anecdotal medicine. "Let Mummy kiss it and make it well" conveys the principle, if not the complete methodology pioneered by Giacomo. His ability to rescue women teetering on the brink of the grave remains a model of heroic measures and hands-on procedure . . .

"We continued to pass such nights as these for weeks, and I had the pleasure of seeing her thoroughly cured. I would have doubtless have married her, if something most unexpected had not happened to me towards the end of the month."

What happened was the Inquisition threw him into prison, for practicing magic.

So, should the Casanovan think of himself as a walking E.R., providing his own variation on C.P.R. to any lass he meets who complains that her doctor has cold hands and heart to match? Perhaps not. But should he come upon a pretty lady already languishing in bed, as some conventional quack's patient, the Casanovan does have the medical precedent for initiating the operation whose anaesthetic is the breath of love.

∿ Thighs

Rare sightings, these were, for the bird watchers of Casanova's time. Relatively modest female garb, and the absence of women's soccer leagues, did not favour the male's seeing the female leg as more than a means of locomotion, hopefully bedward.

When, therefore, chance did present a vista of upper limb, it was an exhilarating experience: ". . . as the veil was short, I could see the bases and almost the frieze of two marble columns; and at this sight I gave a voluptuous cry . . ."

Trust the sensitive Giacomo to see a woman's thighs to be as awe-inspiring as the pillars of the Parthenon. For us today, so accustomed to the spectacle at the public beach or private pool, familiarity has bred, if not contempt, at least a degree of *déjà vu*.

There is very little of his girl-friend's physiognomy that the Casanovan has not already seen, before he sees all of it. Consequently he is less likely to utter "a voluptuous cry" when she drops her shorts.

Titillation, in Casanova's time, relied heavily on the first syllable. [*See* BREASTS]

However, he did avail himself of thighs as a means of introduction — to Mlle. Anne de Roman-Coupier:

"At supper, her napkin fell down and in returning it I pressed her thigh amorously and could not detect the slightest displeasure on her face."

The old Dropped Napkin Gambit. Probably the riskiest opening in the whole arsenal of the mating chess game. Especially at a dinner table where cutlery is at hand, should the lady react unfavourably. The distinction between pressing the thigh "amorously" and gross groping lies very much in the mind of the thigh's owner. Also, there is always the hazard of fondling a table-leg by mistake.

Many foraging Casanovas go to the theatre — as did the maestro — or to cinemas in hopes that the close seating will facilitate thigh contact with an attractive woman adjoining. This may be more subtle than deliberately spilling his popcorn into her lap, and trying to claw it back with the cup, yet in daylight the woman's thigh may prove to evoke a marble column less than a fireplug.

Today, as an indicator of romantic interest, it is not unusual for a woman to leap at a man, wrapping her thighs around his waist and kissing him passionately on the mouth. If this ever happened to Jacques, the overture was not recorded in his memoirs. The Casanova must draw his own conclusions — on the basis of what he has observed on WWF RAW.

∼ Tizzy

"She wept and stormed alternately."

The predictable response to every Casanovan, from the woman he has — in her judgment — wronged.

The first time he is confronted by feminine fury, a man is tempted to argue his case, as if the situation called for the exercise of reason. Jacques cautions:

"It is never of any use to try to convince people in distress that they are wrong, for one may only do harm, while if they are left to themselves they soon feel that they have been unjust, and are grateful to the person who let them exhaust their grief without any contradiction . . ."

The voice of experience. Casanova had dozens of hysterical women whom he refrained from arguing with, and who later appreciated his letting them enjoy full rein to their reaction to his behaving like a prick.

The soft answer not only turneth away wrath but stalleth possible legal action.

To protest merely invites being hit, with whatever object comes to hand — car-seat cushion . . . bedlamp . . . pool cue. And the Casanovan requires utmost self-discipline not to hit back. Instead, he maintains the air of a martyr to circumstances beyond his control. He absorbs the slings and arrows of the outraged Ms. with the patience of a St. Sebastian.

Today, the most common cause of the female tizzy is her lover's balking at COMMITMENT. He must expect to listen (nodding sadly) to the catalogue of reasons why he is unable to commit: clinical paranoia about marriage . . . altarphobia . . . latent homosexuality . . . All, alas, too true.

Even more audible can be a woman's reaction to her lover's announcement that henceforth he is going to be unavailable for social engagements because he:

    (a) has had dental work that left him impotent, or

    (b) just realized that he prefers young boys, or

    (c) is joining the French Foreign Legion.

Sound reasons, all. And futile. More practical is to let the tizzy thrower exhaust her rage, assured that the tears and tantrum provide a physical and mental catharsis for a woman, far less harmful to health than the male's phlegm. His being the strong, silent type is the cardiologist's bread and butter.

And, to avoid the major eruption that can bury him under verbal lava, he should ever remember:

Never, the dumper be,
always seem the dumpee.

～ Touching

Casanova was not one to rush to judgement, in appraising the structural qualities of his latest project. One caress (i.e. touching) is worth more than the other four senses combined, to validate a figure.

Whenever possible, Jacques touched with his lips. One of the great losses to romance has been the courtly custom of the gentleman's kissing the lady's hand. By subtle pressure of fingers on palm, the gentleman conveyed the promise of even more labial contact to come, as well as his getting a good look at the rings on her fingers, should these enter into his planning.

Far too many Casanovans confuse affective touching with groping, the gross enterprise that triggers so many charges of sexual harassment. Women do not respond well to a rugby tackle around the waist. Nor are shoulders the erogenous zone that some men — hearty huggers — hope them to be.

What about playing footsie? Casanova does not appear to have been a great believer in pedal nuzzling. When a woman is wearing expensive pumps, being probed by someone's Nike sneaker contributes little to her rapture.

In John Steinbeck's play *Of Mice and Men,* rancher Curly wears a vaselined sheath on his finger, to protect his wife from the rough touch of a man of the soil. Only mildly endearing. But the Casanovan will do well to remember that for Jacques his lips had much to say before he uttered a word.

Needless to say, he did not wear a MOUSTACHE. Tickling is the kind of touching best restricted to family cats and fat aunts.

～ Tough Love

Casanova has been to a party, in Moscow, one to which his current mistress was not invited . . .

"I got home, and, fortunately for myself, escaped the bottle which Zaira flung at my head, and which would infallibly have killed me if it had hit me . . ." (Casanova had great reflexes, essential to his type of social life.) "She threw herself on the ground, and began to strike it with her forehead . . ."

Sound familiar? Remind you of homecoming? Post office party?

Yes, Hell hath no fury like a woman who thinks her partner has enjoyed an orgy without her. Casanova's idea of a sedative: a knuckle sandwich. "In Russia beating is a matter of necessity, for words have no force whatever. A servant, mistress or courtesan understands nothing but the lash . . ."

The direct approach to problem solving.

What is perhaps more relevant to the Casanovan today, Casanova's rationale for the effect of repeated beatings of his fourteen-year-old blintze:

"My master has not sent me away, but beaten me; therefore he loves me, and I ought to be attached to him."

Even though it is a statistical fact that women initiate domestic violence as often as men, today it is the male who gets the chance to experience the suspension and interior décor of the paddy wagon. *Autre temps, autres moeurs.* So, either take your mistress to the party or remove all the bottles from the bedroom. Even when visiting Moscow.

∽ Trade-Ins

"Before I left Russia, Rinaldi, the seventy-year-old architect of the Queen pleaded with me to sell him Zaira, with whom he had fallen in love. But I gave joy to the heart of the beautiful young women by returning her to her parents, so that they could re-sell her to Rinaldi."

It's the little gestures that count. Like, making your significant other feel good about being returned to her family for re-marketing.

This kind of heart-warming transaction is less feasible today for the Casanovan, because women have found careers other than domestic love slave — a pity, but education is flawed.

What is interesting about Casanova's business dealing of the dusky Zaira is that more and more North American men are seeking women in Russia, or India, via the Internet. Object, matrimony, but sometimes the service falls short of the altar.

The point is, because women in lands that are less economically favored than the West are desperate for escape, they seem to offer a better deal for American men looking for a sexy housekeeper with a feeble grasp on the English language. The only catch is that, unlike Casanova, the owner cannot return his buy to her family for resale.

This is just one of many ways in which Casanova had a more rewarding sex life than the average computer owner. The only laptop he had to trust was his own. Which conveyed personal messages for short distance but with sensational effect.

Today's shrunken market for previously owned lovers helps to explain why so many men have transferred their love life from women to other moving objects. Like, trucks. Knowing that he can, if necessary, trade in his beloved Ford 150 — the pickup not found in a bar— enhances the owner's relationship with this trusty travelling companion.

Casanova would have loved to have had one. Besides, of course, his utility Zaira — loaded, immac, b.o.

⮞ Transport

Casanova was the ultimate travelling man, love's road warrior.

His means of travel were as various as the era allowed. (He never flew.) When we consider the staggering number of his sexual conquests, we have to be awed to imagine what Casanova would have wrought had he had access to the automobile. Our mobile boudoir.

On the other hand, Casanova usually rode as a fellow passenger in carriage or jitney, freeing up both hands that otherwise might have been distracted by driving. [See GONDOLAS]

Despite the variety of his means of transportation, he did not establish a lasting relationship with a horse. Faithful or otherwise. His first serious encounter with the saddle was aboard a horse he had stolen, in a hasty escape from the law. All his subsequent trips on horseback were also in emergencies only. No horse got to know him intimately, nor he it. The conveyance that kept John Wayne a strong, silent man short on women: a no-go for the amorous Venetian. He reserved the equestrian position for his women. And almost certainly enjoyed more sex than the Lone Ranger.

But the most important factor in Casanova's choice of transport — and an example to every aspiring Casanovan — was that it took him *where he wanted to go*. Sometimes his ship would be blown off-course, or even stranded, but it was an act of God, not wife. He had no one nagging "Look at the map, stupid! We're headed in the wrong direction!"

⌒ Travel

"He travels fastest who travels alone." Speed was not a factor, when Casanova was travelling, unless he was being pursued by representatives of the law. Normally he preferred to have company — female, of course — either en route or at wayside inns where the maid service would help him find travel broadening.

Casanova had a sex drive that got him more miles to the gal.

Yet he usually travelled with a strong sense of final destination. Ramble, he didn't. A person who toured not only the cities but the wilds of Europe and Asia Minor might be expected to mention, somewhere in his memoirs, the beauty of nature. But it was the nature of beauty (feminine) that fascinated Casanova.

He had no inkling that his work was about to be overtaken by romanticism. He had no time for trees. He was too busy sizing up the latest girl he was travelling with — the ideal situation for the Casanovan. Women *expect* romance when journeying alone, and away from home. For many their moral scruples are shored up by the presence of parents, a husband, a dog that gets nasty when jealous. But put a woman alone, in a foreign city, and she will be severely disappointed if she has to sleep by herself. (Most hotel beds are queen-size, which just rubs it in.)

Morals don't travel well.

Yet *premeditated* travel-for-sex — to the Club Med, for instance — usually bombs. Female guests and staff recognize desperation when they see it. The Casanovan will lose out to a busboy.

◈ Venetian

". . . I found her charming in bed. I had not enjoyed the Venetian vices for nearly eight years, and she was a beauty before whom Praxitiles would have bent the knee."

Casanova does not detail the Venetian vices, leaving — as always — some specifics to our imagination and what we remember from watching Fellini films (including his *Casanova*).

One can only conjecture as to how strong was the influence of his Venetian home environment on the matchless record of raunchy romance set by this sexual phenomenon. The very name, Venice, has the same parentage — Venus — as some of our common (*very* common) words: *venereal, venery,* as well as that anatomical Everest, *mons veneris.*

V is the second-most sexy letter of our alphabet, only S being more suggestive.

It follows that a city like Toronto (T) is unlikely to be competitive with Venice, as a nurturing source of the devout Casanovan. Vancouver has the right initial, but its vices have never been seen as distinctive. Being able to ski and play tennis on the same day leaves little time for creating sexual variations that identify the resident while travelling abroad.

The word vices, too, starts with the letter that is all cleavage. V. Which also inhabits the name Casanovan. But how else does its bearer acquire the amatory skills of the son or daughter of Venice?

Regrettably, the usual guided tour of Venus's city does not include a viewing of its historical vices. British tourists (especially women) have been traipsing across the Bridge of Sighs for scores of years, without picking up much of anything except Murano glass brandy snifters.

So, the apprentice Casanovan who has been born in Turkey Weed, Saskatchewan, must just accept the fact that, vice-wise, he has much to learn and no canals to cool him off. But who said that life was fair?

⟍ Virginity

"Irrespective of birth, beauty and wit, which was the principal merit of my new conquest, prejudice was there to enhance a hundredfold my felicity, for she was a vestal: it was forbidden fruit, and who does not know that, from Eve to our days, it was the fruit which has always appeared the most delicious! I was on the point of encroaching upon the rights of an all-powerful husband . . ."

All-powerful husbands being a rare commodity today, the Casanovan is less likely to be poaching on their rights. But it is significant that what made the "fruit" delicious to Jacques was that it was "forbidden." (Madeleine being a nun.) Stolen sweets are sweeter. And well worth pinching. As with the delicious Raton, who merely feigned virginity, without being particularly vestal:

". . . I was well satisfied and, not caring much for maidenheads, I rewarded her as if I had been the first to bite at the cherry."

Casanova does almost as much fruit-picking, lifetime, as the average Okanagan orchardist. And sometimes does not consider it to be a challenge worthy of the trouble:

". . . for it is often a matter of some difficulty to pluck the first flower; and the price which most men put on this little trifle is founded more on egotism than any feeling of pleasure."

Today, most girls have had the flower picked before they even graduate from high-school, though the recent abstinence movement may affect the Casanovan till he goes to college. At whatever stage he encounters the hymen — which can be considerably less yielding than a Bing — the reduced chance of also picking up an STD may be offset by collateral damage to the conscience. (Does this mean she will expect me to marry her?)

What if the embryonic Casanovan is himself a virgin? This is a situation almost too awful to contemplate. People (especially women) can be put off sex for years, as a result of this bloody collision that is not covered by insurance.

But it can happen. How a guy is to lose his virginity, without violating a maid or having it off with a hooker, is a procedure for which no properly diagrammed manual exists. A man never discusses it. Like the war veteran, he refuses to recall the battle.

Luckily, we are having more cases of female schoolteachers seducing an adolescent boy in their class. If this trend comes too late for the Casanovan, at least he can hope that a more liberal education will bless his bastard son.

❧ Virtue

"I have always had a profligate life, and have not always been very delicate in the choice of means to gratify my passions, but even amidst my vices I was always a passionate lover of virtue."

The retired roué is confessing to a passion less evident when he was young.

But in fact this celebrated libertine did have virtue to counterbalance his womanizing: "Benevolence, especially, has always had a great charm for me, and I have never failed to exercise it unless restrained by the desire for vengeance — a vice which has always had a controlling influence on my actions."

True enough. No one could fault Casanova for being mean-spirited. He spared no expense, in cash or courtesies, to please a lady. He hosted lavish dinner parties that he couldn't afford. He was quick to come to the rescue of a damsel in distress. Sometimes she just exchanged one distress for another, but at least he added variety.

Casanova had the virtue of being a simple man. He simply wanted love. Some men — those unworthy of the name of Casanovans — in seducing women are motivated by other than the joy of sex. Having failed at projects that required them to get out of bed, they settle for the one that gets them back *into* bed.

The person who reads *The History of My Life* just to winkle out the bawdy bits will miss the array of virtues that contributed as much to Casanova's success with women as his amatory prowess. Paramount among them: his HONESTY.

Granted, Casanova was a chronic and compulsive gambler — not considered a virtue outside Vegas city limits. He gambled with everything, including his life, as was shown by his record of deadly duels, with sword or pistol at a few paces. But he was ever a gentleman in solicitous aid to the rival he had grievously wounded. This Italian did not subscribe to the Sicilian belief that revenge is a dish best eaten cold.

The message: the Casanovan, to succeed, needs more than the roving eye. And no matter how large his other organ, he shall fail without the generous heart.

꩜ Voyeurism

Is the flip side of exhibitionism. Jacques is able to indulge in both kinds of kinky sex, when his beloved Madeleine — nun *extraordinaire* — asks him to allow her other, senior lover to watch, from a peephole in the closet, while she and Casanova make love. Ever ready to take the broad view, he agrees to participate in the private spectacle . . .

"If a feeling of modesty does not deter you from shewing yourself tender, loving, and full of amorous ardour with me in his presence, how could I be ashamed, when, on the contrary, I ought to feel proud of myself?"

As a means of building self-esteem, this method is not apt to be offered to the average Casanovan. Even if he has found success as a male porn film star, he loses amateur status such as that enjoyed by the Master. Who tells his versatile mistress:

". . . most men object to any witness in those moments, but those who cannot give any good reasons for their repugnance must have in their nature something of the cat."

This is one of the rare references to felines in the memoirs. Casanova never had a four-legged pet of any kind, being too much of a gypsy to look after any animal but himself. He has, however, obviously noticed that — unlike dogs, which are shameless exhibitionists in their sexual encounters — cats are secretive, night-time lovers, despite the occasional ecstatic yowl.

Had the video camera been available in his time, would Casanova have used it to create a voyeuristic photo archive to complement his collection of incandescent correspondence? Probably not. Unless, of course, the lady suggested it, brought her own props and signed an agreement not to market the video without his sharing the proceeds.

As for watching some other guy have sex with Casanova's inamorata, he demurred: ". . . I would go away, for I could not remain a quiet spectator."

For Giacomo, love-making was not a spectator sport. Like ice curling, it is a game for the participants. If the Casanovan is unable to enjoy it without the roar of the crowd, he should be looking at some other physical contest, that dispenses with clothing. Pro wrestling comes to mind.

~ Wedding Present

What to give to your girl friend on the eve of her marrying some-one else?

This problem is a common one among Casanovans who like to be remembered fondly, if at all. The conventional wedding present — a set of silver finger-bowls — doesn't seem appropriate, in the cir-cumstances. For our role model, however, it was no problem:

"She [Mariuccia] told me that she was to be married on the eve of Shrove Tuesday, and she arranged to spend four hours with me on the Sunday before her wedding."

Casanova pledged his own brand of troth: "I promise you that when you leave me you will be in such a state that the caresses of your husband will not hurt you."

And at 7 a.m. of the Sabbath, Casanova presents Mariuccia with the four hours of bliss, gift-wrapped. "After the sixth song we were weary, though not satiated. We parted with tears, swearing to love each other forever after, as brother and sister. She promised that if the morning resulted in a child, it would be named after me."

Now, *that* is a wedding present. One that can be appreciated as much by the donor as by the recipient. It is more blessed to give, etc.

The carping critic will point out that giving the bride-to-be four hours of sensationally orgasmic pleasure might prejudice the chances of the groom as a hard — very hard — act to follow. But the wise head will judge that a woman has no difficulty in recalling the ecstasy bestowed by a previous lover, while being utilized by her husband. It is why she closes her eyes. And avoids moaning a name other than "Sweetie."

It should be noted that, by combining his wedding present with the celebration of Easter, Casanova put several eggs in one basket, with every chance of their being fertilized.

To attempt to emulate this bridal gifting — somewhat more personal and memorable than that suggested by Miss Manners — may be beyond the scope of the Casanovan. Unless of course he receives an engraved invitation, requesting the honour of his presence . . .

⌘ Wind

The wind in the pillows. The first time that the Casanovan encounters the passion-gassing flatulence he should recall Giacomo's hilarious account of his defeat by woman's ultimate weapon. (Ignored by The Geneva Convention)

". . . at the very first jump a disturbing noise somewhat cooled my ardour, the more so that the young girl covered her face with her hands. However, encouraging her with a loving kiss, I began again. But now a report, louder even than the first, distracted me. I tried to continue; there came a third, a fourth, and, to make a long matter short, the spectacle was as if an orchestra conductor was beating out the time and was being obeyed with precision by an instrument which compensated for the monotony of its tone by its powerful assault on another of the senses."

Casanova broke up in laughter. The girl fled, mortified. The harmonics of sex cannot tolerate the addition of a loose bassoon.

For the virginal female, the synchronized fart is as effective as a chastity belt. For which there is no key.

Sexually experienced women who suffer from The Curse That Has No Name will usually warn a new lover before the action becomes too squally . . .

"I'm awfully sorry, but I pass gas during intercourse."

What, if any, is the Casanovan's appropriate response to this warning?

"That's okay, honey, I live with an old dog."

Nothing really suits the situation. Turning up the stereo may muffle the eruptions but, given the vigorous exertions of sex, to stop inhaling could compromise the Casanovan's chances of surviving what ought to be a healthful exercise. Muses Jacques:

"I am sure the young girl was indebted to that singular weakness for the strength of her virtue and most likely, if it were common to all the fair sex, the whole world would be far lonelier than it is."

Indeed. An ill wind that blows nobody good.

Conclusion: be suspicious of any over-thirty woman who says she is still a virgin. The reason for her maidenhood may lie less with virtue than with viscera.

⇜ Wine

"Candy/ Is dandy/ But liquor/ Is quicker."

These immortal lines, from Ogden Nash's "Reflections On Icebreaking," express with exquisite precision a guiding principle of Casanova's lubricating the lust. Consider this passage from the memoirs, typical of his myriad accounts of seduction:

"We had an excellent supper and she kept pace with me both in eating and the excellent claret. Not being used to wine, her passions were aroused and her gaiety made her look even more lovely . . ."

With the bottle having broken the ice, his date submits gladly to his ardent kisses. But she passes out in his embrace . . .

"The claret numbed her senses, and I could tell that she was having a dream . . ." Ever adaptable, Casanova provides the appropriate physical accompaniment to her dreaming.

Now, the purist may complain that using alcohol to help a maid overcome any sexual inhibitions is an unsporting tactic. But on the other hand, even the most cloistered nun has seen a priest or two get giggly on the sacramental wine.

Everyone needs an excuse for being naughty.

Casanova understood this truth as it applied to women. He knew that the difference between plying a girl with alcohol (bad), and liberating her libido with wine (good) lies in the quality of the drink. The operative word, above: "the *excellent* claret." No cheap plonk for Jacques. Nothing but the best. A woman knows when the dinner wine has cost her suitor an arm and a leg, and is disposed to make it up to his remaining appendages.

A mug of beer, a shot-glass of whiskey, and a glass of wine are said to contain the same amount of alcohol. But the effect on a woman is in no-wise comparable. Despite the liberation of women and the shortage of virgin nuns, the Casanovan will do well to remember that the Master set the standard for romantic encounter, with the cherry yielding to the grape.

To the best of his biographers' knowledge, Casanova rarely hated himself in the morning. And that, surely, exonerates the fine dinner wine.

⮚ Wisdom

"A young girl learns deeper lessons from nature than we men can acquire with all our experience." Casanova is reflecting on the unfair advantage that women have over men, and that makes victims of us all.

Feminine INTUITION. That fearsome power is one reason why men are readily duped. When we speak of an "old fool" we invariably refer to a male geezer, trying to put the hit on a woman many years his junior. In his sixties, Casanova too was tempted, by a pretty harlequin he met at a Trieste carnival:

"Naturally, I fell in love with her, but as I was her senior by thirty years, and had begun my addresses in a tone of fatherly affection, a feeling of shame prevented my disclosing to her the real state of my heart."

This aging libertine knew when to say "when." And wisely so.

Wisdom may be defined as the product of intelligence conditioned by experience. Casanova's I.Q. — had there been any way of measuring it beyond knowing how to tie one's shoelaces — would have been in the genius range. As for experiences, few men have enjoyed such a wide scope of adventures, amatory and otherwise. Thus, as a senior, he was able to avoid the foolishness of many older men bent on sex with a much younger woman — usually a high-rolling blond with a deep affection for diamonds, yachts and BMWs.

"As for the pleasures of love, I enjoyed them in moderation, taking care of my purse and of my health."

Conclusion: elderly Casanovan is an oxymoron. It is only the Don Juan — the libertine who basically hates women — who is apt to appear in our newspaper's society gossip column, photographed leering in tandem with a bimbo young enough to be his daughter and smart enough to exploit a sex drive that spends a lot of time in neutral.

The Casanovan may shudder at the prospect of having his lusty libido reduced, by time, to "a tone of fatherly affection." He need not, however, fear becoming prematurely wise. His natural sexual impulse ensures the triumph of folly over sagacity. And women will love him for it.

⟶ Wit

"Beauty without wit offers love nothing but the material enjoyment of its physical charms, whilst witty ugliness captivates by the charms of the mind, and at last fulfils all the desires of the man it has captivated."

Profoundly true. Also true: the Casanovan will be all too likely to settle for the "physical charms" of beauty, even though they fail to sustain him long-term. Casanova himself opted, quite frequently, for the material charms of teenage beauties while, intellectually, he recognized that a homely woman of wit would be more likely to fulfil him when the bloom was off the rose.

Thus do our appetites betray our digestion.

Women have a name for the witless sex kitten: *bimbo.* (a.k.a. *Barbie Doll*) No doubt the currency of "bimbo" among women — especially feminists — does reflect a certain amount of pussy envy. They rightly deplore the fact that, though beauty is only skin deep, the subcutaneous virtues of a woman are not what attract a man, assuming that he has at least 10-percent vision.

Complicating matters is that good looks do not necessarily *preclude* wit. Some beautiful women deliberately downplay their wit, lest it spook a man they find to be a "hunk."

Their dress can be more revealing than their conversation.

It will then come as a devastating shock to the trainee Casanovan when the gorgeous chick he assumes to have little between the ears but erotic ideas suddenly, and with a volley of sharp wit, dumps him. He should have read his Oscar Wilde.

The plain woman, in contrast, unable to win attention with surface features, will be motivated to use such wit as she has available. Which of course has a longer shelf-life than bosoms and butts. The Casanovan who squires a truly ugly woman of charming wit will find himself the cynosure of comely women. He will have to beat them off with a swizzle-stick.

Beauty is only relative. Viz, in an Alaskan village where there is only one woman, she will look unspeakably lovely to the entire male population. But a woman of wit can hold her own on the beach at the Cannes film festival of flawless flesh.

The Casanovan ought to keep this truth in mind, even as he inevitably ignores it.

⟨≋⟩ Women

Contrary to common belief among men, the word woman does not derive from the fusing of *woe* and *man*. It comes from the OE *wif-man,* or wife of a human being. No wonder women (in English) have had an uphill battle to free themselves from that first, subservient syllable.

The French woman has fared better, as *la femme.* No relation to *l'homme*. Two distinct genders, from the get-go. Woman or wife, *une femme* serves us all.

Especially all of Casanova. Our Venetian playboy sampled females of most of the civilized world, and was unequivocal about his preference for the mademoiselle or madame. French women were free spirits who could take him on, or under. Whether it was a serving wench or Madame Pompadour that he was beguiling, she had full confidence in her femininity.

The eighteenth-century *grande dame* of France could be as financially and socially successful as today's career woman, without coercion by computer. Her boudoir served as *salon* for the wits and wantons on whom the guillotine had yet to cast its shadow. (Casanova, by the way, had nothing good to say about the French Revolution. "That popular effervescence has disgusted me," the old rake sniffs in his memoirs. All those lovely, elegant necks lost to the kiss of a blade so brutal!)

Today, the Casanovan must try to deal with, so to speak, a broad range of women. The North American variety may well be overtly aggressive sexually, if she fancies him, and if his jeans offer promise. Desperate single moms lie in ambush behind every school reunion, any beach log, in adjoining plane seats.

Above all, in every woman today may lurk a closet feminist, eager to avenge the wifman. Caveat raptor!

⚒ Your Memoirs

Is it premature for the Casanovan — of any age — to be thinking about writing his own memoirs? Ans: gentlemen, start your hard drives!

It is never too soon for the sexually hyper-active man to begin making notes. Your memory may be the first thing to burn out, if you get really lucky.

Casanova seems to have enjoyed an elephantine memory — seconded by a robust imagination — to help him eventually chronicle his adventures, since he was travelling too light to keep memoranda and file copies.

In this regard, keeping a journal may be useful to the memoirist who wants to include a few facts with the fiction of his romantic affairs. Such a diary need not be devoted entirely to sexual encounters, and may actually act as a stimulus if, after a year, it has failed to mention any event more erotic than his nightmare about being gang-raped by insatiable aliens with big breasts.

Chances are, the Casanovan's own father is writing *his* memoirs right this minute, leaving out the episode of his knocking up the girl whose big brother — the rugby player — persuaded him to marry her.

Writing his memoirs is one of the major compulsions of the older man. He wants to leave something on paper, other than t.p. For this reason the young Casanova disciple will strive to live each day as though it was not only his last but of possible interest to a publisher, later on.

Like the memoirs of Casanova, yours need not be entirely concerned with sex. But a chronicle whose motif is essentially sexless, such as that of a Canadian politician, will probably need to be published by a vanity press unless the memoirist has had more than one term as prime minister.

⤳ Zilch

It would be nice if the candidate for Casanovism could picture the paradigm of promiscuity as comfortably retired, enjoying his own cozy cottage, warmed by his significant other plus civilized grandchildren.

Don't eat that, Elmer.

The facts of Casanova's life in old age give us a picture of a crabby, whining codger owning zilch except his memories.

He sank to the level of begging for employment by the same tribunal of the Inquisition that sent him into The Leads prison. Working for them as a spy. As when reporting on a painting academy where nudes posed for portraits and visitors were welcome. As Levinson observes: "The eagle became a stool pigeon."

After that jejune job petered out, Casanova grumbled around the bleak library of Count Waldstein, in dreary Dux Castle, northern Bohemia, writing letters and of course the monumental memoirs.

The message for the would-be Casanovan: unless you plan to die young — and it is an option worth offering to the gods — you really need to have some occupation besides bedding women and betting on cards. We all die alone, but it is the wretched years while we teeter ere hopping the twig that may make the Casanovan question the wisdom of his never having learned a trade . . . or married a nice girl . . . or at least invested in sound real estate.

He who sows wild oats only, reaps a thin crop.

With his swashbuckling lifestyle — fighting duels, making love to married women, eating out to excess — Casanova was lucky to live as long as he did. Or was he? He had no way of knowing that his massive memoirs would qualify as one of the classics of eighteenth-century literature. Grown old, he might have been happier had he had a good-natured missus to bring him a cup of tea, and rub the back that he compromised with too much indoor sport.

In short, Casanovism. Total dedication to the pleasure principle, with emphasis on the opposite sex, may not be indicated after all.

This is particularly true if — unlike *the* Casanova — his disciple has missed the point: women are to be *loved*. He who has intercourse merely to relieve sexual tension is like the person whose only interest in food is to satisfy hunger. Both are a bit gross. Women are fascinating creatures, usually seeking more than sex. They are the gourmets of copulation, whereas most men are into fast food.

The wolf misses all the nuances of romance that made every love affair memorable for Giacomo, because he wasn't trying to squeeze it in between soccer practices.

Lord Byron — no mean libertine himself — wrote: "Man's love is of man's life a thing apart, / 'Tis woman's whole existence." To-day's woman has narrowed the gap of need for a man's love, thanks to the resurrection of Sappho, plus the technological break-through of the vibrator, and golf links for ladies.

Another new reality to make the Casanovan's sex life more complicated than that of the average fruit fly: a new generation of women — to the consternation of the vintage feminists — is reported to be making waves in the Sea of Discord:

The neo-feminist.

This brash young thing has taken a long look at her older sisters in emancipation from the patriarchal family, and noticed that the even playing field has proved to be crabgrass. Having it all — career . . . kids . . . a male helpmate eager and happy to forego the hockey game in favour of vacuuming the dog — has been found to be a flawed concept.

Total gender equality has been no guarantee of happiness for either sex. Especially if the hired nanny fashions a kid who views his or her parents as home furnishing, readily replaced by a computer play station.

As bonding, it's been Crazy Glue.

So, now the younger woman is seeking to restore her role as a homemaker, perhaps postponing another career in order to enjoy the satisfaction of being a full-time Mom.

What is the Casanovan to make of this? Every hour that this woman spends with her children means less time that she will be sitting in a bar, or schussing down the slope, or taking her rightful place at a pool table, where the Casanovan has the opportunity to catch her eye and take a cue. Instead, she is ensconced in her home office, flirting with the Internet, a rival more formidable than any Giacomo ever had to deal with.

Thus the would-be Casanovan faces different criteria for seducing a nineteen-year-old university freshette, her forty-year-old unwed mother, and her understandably alcoholic grannie.

This frightening development has occurred in the time it has taken to write this book. Which makes it difficult to assess the Casanovan's chances of finding sexual fulfillment by helping Moms push swings in playgrounds. Or by becoming a PC repairman, in order to get noticed by cyberwoman.

However, this rapidly-evolving confusion of gender roles does not necessarily invalidate the preceding pages' gospel according to Casanova. A woman is ever a woman. And still susceptible to the advances of the man who truly loves women — preferably one at a time, but with mind open to exceptional occasions.

Good hunting!

ABOUT THE AUTHOR

Eric Nicol has authored 34 books (three of them Leacock Medal winners), written seven plays for the legitimate stage, and fathered three children, also legitimate.

If questioned about his qualifications to discuss the memoirs of the world's greatest lover — Jacques Casanova — Nicol points out that his maternal great-grandfather was also Italian. Hence the probability of inheriting sexy genes. Also Nicol admits to his being very fond of women, as his favourite gender, and wouldn't mind having more experience with them as a result of publication of this book.

Meanwhile he is married, to novelist Mary Razzell, and is interested in breathing.